Sport, Medicine and He

The relationship between sport, medicine and health in our society is becoming increasingly complex. This important and timely study explores this relationship through an analysis of changing political economies, altered perceptions of the body and science's developing contribution to the human condition. Surveying the various ways in which medicine interacts with the world of sport, it examines the changing practices and purposes of sports medicine today.

Drawing on the latest research in the sociology of sport, this book investigates the scientific discourse underlying the promotion of physical activity to reveal the political context in which medical knowledge and public policies emerge. It considers the incongruities between these policies and their attempts to regulate the supply of, and demand for, sports medicine. Through a series of original case studies, this book exposes the social construction of sports medical knowledge and questions the potential for medicine to influence athletes' well-being both positively and negatively.

Sport, Medicine and Health: The medicalization of sport? provides valuable insights for all students and scholars interested in sports medicine, sports policy, public health and the sociology of sport.

Dominic Malcolm is a Reader in the Sociology of Sport at Loughborough University, UK.

Routledge Research in Sport, Culture and Society

Sport, Medicine and Health

The Medicalization of Sport?

Dominic Malcolm

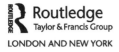

LONDON AND NEW YORK

First published 2017
by Routledge
2 Park Square, Milton Park, Abingdon, Oxon OX14 4RN

and by Routledge
711 Third Avenue, New York, NY 10017

First issued in paperback 2018

Routledge is an imprint of the Taylor & Francis Group, an informa business

British Library Cataloguing-in-Publication Data
A catalogue record for this book is available from the British
Library

Library of Congress Cataloging in Publication Data
Names: Malcolm, Dominic, 1969– author.
Title: Sport, medicine and health : the medicalization of sport? /
Dominic Malcolm.
Description: Milton Park, Abingdon, Oxon ; New York, NY :
Routledge, 2016. |
Series: Routledge research in sport, culture and society ; 69
| Includes bibliographical references and index.
Identifiers: LCCN 2016028563| ISBN 9781138826458 (hbk)
| ISBN 9781315573931 (ebk)
Subjects: LCSH: Sport medicine. | Sports–Sociological aspects.
Classification: LCC RC1210 .M265 2016 | DDC 617.1/027–dc23
LC record available at https://lccn.loc.gov/2016028563

ISBN 13: 978-1-138-31765-9 (pbk)
ISBN 13: 978-1-138-82645-8 (hbk)

Typeset in Sabon
by Wearset Ltd, Boldon, Tyne and Wear

Contents

Acknowledgements

The book is the culmination of about 15 years of researching and writing in this area (see Appendix 1). I am particularly indebted to the many people who have given up their time to complete questionnaires and/or volunteer their thoughts in interviews. I am also very grateful to the various colleagues with whom I have collaborated along the way. In chronological order of their initial influence on this work I would like to thank Ivan Waddington, Martin Roderick, Ken Sheard, Stuart Smith, Andrea Scott, Parissa Safai, Louise Mansfield, Lauren Sherar, Mike Morgan, Mark Orme, Emma Pullen and Patrick Wheeler. Most of all though, I would like to thank my family for supporting me in my work, for listening to my random thoughts along the way and, ultimately, just for being there for me.

Abbreviations

ABA	Amateur Boxing Association
ACC	American College of Cardiology
ACPSM	Association of Chartered Physiotherapists in Sports Medicine
ACSM	American College of Sports Medicine
AFL	Australian Football League
AHA	American Heart Association
AMA	American Medical Association
AMRC	Academy of Medical Royal Colleges
APA	Australian Physiotherapy Association
APCPA	All-Party Commission on Physical Activity
BASEM	British Association of Sport and Exercise Medicine
BASM	British Association of Sport and Medicine
BATS	British Association of Trauma in Sport
BBBC	British Board of Boxing Control
BHF	British Heart Foundation
BJSM	British Journal of Sports Medicine
BMA	British Medical Association
BOA	British Olympic Association
CAMs	Complementary and Alternative Medicines
CAS	Court of Arbitration for Sport
CASM	Canadian Academy of Sport Medicine
CASS	Canadian Association of Sports Sciences
CHD	Chronic Heart Disease
CISG	Concussion in Sport Guidelines
COPD	Chronic Obstructive Pulmonary Disorder
CPD	Continuing Professional Development
CRY	Cardiac Risk in the Young
CSP	Chartered Society of Physiotherapy
CTE	Chronic Traumatic Encephalopathy
DÄB	Deutscher Ärztebund zur Förderung der Leibesügungen (German Medical Association for the Advancement of Physical Activities)

DNH	Department of National Heritage
DoH	Department of Health
DtM	Designed to Move
ECG	Electrocardiogram
ECHO	Echocardiogram
EiM	Exercise is Medicine
EM	Emergency Medicine
ESC	European Society of Cardiology
FA	Football Association
FIFA	Fédération Internationale de Football Associations
FIMS	Fédération Internationale de Médecine Sportive
FSEM	Faculty of Sport and Exercise Medicine
GMC	General Medical Council
HCM	Hypertrophic Cardiomyopathy
HPC	Health Professions Council
IAAF	International Amateur Athletics Federation
IABSEM	Intercollegiate Academic Board of Sport and Exercise Medicine
IIHF	International Ice Hockey Federation
IOC	International Olympic Committee
IRB	International Rugby Board
ISM	Institute of Sports Medicine
LOC	Loss of Consciousness
LOCOG	London Organising Committee of the Olympic and Paralympic Games
MDTs	Multidisciplinary Teams
MRC	Medical Research Council
MSK	Musculoskeletal
mTBI	mild Traumatic Brain Injury
NBA	National Basketball Association
NCAA	National Collegiate Athletic Association
NFL	National Football League
NGBs	National Governing Bodies
NHL	National Hockey League
NHS	National Health Service
NOC	National Olympic Committee
NPH	New Public Health
NRL	National Rugby League
PAHP	Physical Activity Health Promotion
PEA	Physical Education Association
PFA	Professional Footballers Association
PHE	Public Health England
PR	Pulmonary Rehabilitation
RCP	Royal College of Physicians

RTP	Return To Play
SCAT	Sports Concussion Assessment Tool
SCD	Sudden Cardiac Death
SEM	Sport and Exercise Medicine
SMSCC	Sport Medicine and Science Council of Canada
SRI	Sport-Related Injury
UEFA	Union of European Football Associations
UKAD	United Kingdom Anti-Doping Agency
UKADIS	United Kingdom Association of Doctors in Sports
USOC	United States Olympic Committee
WHO	World Health Organization

Chapter 1

Sport, medicine and health

An introduction

This book explores the complex and contradictory relationships between sport, medicine and health. It stems from the observation that while currently there is considerable evidence that sport is undergoing medicalization – the process whereby 'a problem is defined in medical terms, defined using medical language, understood through the adoption of a medical framework, or "treated" with a medical intervention' (Conrad 2007: 5) – the development is multi-linear and at times contradictory to sport as an institution and athletes as a population exhibiting a high degree of relative autonomy. The book evokes a re-consideration of two socially pervasive ideas, namely: that sports participation is a fundamental and necessary part of a healthy lifestyle (the sport–health ideology); and that elite sport rationally exploits science and medicine in the pursuit of competitive success. It does so by drawing on a wide range of empirical research based on interviews, questionnaire surveys and documentary sources and through a more rigorous and systematic cross-fertilization of the sociologies of sport and medicine/health and illness than has hitherto been undertaken. Underpinned by an Eliasian sociological perspective it is an ambitious attempt to explore these phenomena holistically, via the interaction of their macro, meso and micro manifestations, their societal, institutional and interactional spheres. We begin therefore by sketching the breadth of the contemporary manifestations of this nexus of relationships.

Contemporary manifestations of the medicalization of sport

The medicalization of sport is a global movement. In 2003 the United Nations General Assembly adopted 'Resolution 58/5: Sport as a Means to Promote, Health, Education and Peace', which pronounced that 'Sport and play improve health and well-being, extend life expectancy and reduce the likelihood of several non-communicable diseases.... Regular physical activity and play are essential for physical, mental, psychological and social development' (cited in Safai 2008). In the same year, the World Health

Organization (WHO 2003) published *Health and Development through Physical Activity and Sport*, which identified:

> a new challenge and at the same time a tremendous opportunity for the sports movement as a whole ... [to] contribute uniquely and importantly to the promotion of public health and at the same time strengthen social credibility and accountability of sport.
>
> (Cited in Bloyce and Smith 2009: 112)

In so doing the UN and WHO firmly located sport as part of the traditional domain on medicine.

Following this, the *European Union Physical Activity Guidelines* were approved (European Union 2008), *Developing the European Dimension in Sport* (European Union 2011) positioned sport as fundamental to physical activity health promotion, and WHO (2012) published *Global Recommendations on Physical Activity for Health*. The prevalence of such policies within Europe was illustrated in *Promoting Sport and Enhancing Health in European Union Countries* (WHO 2011). The documentary review underpinning this report identified 130 national policies published within the European Region between 2000 and 2009 (112 from the 27 EU member states). Analysis of a sample of 25 concluded that 'all strategies mentioned health-enhancing physical activity and contained overall goals on participation in sport and physical activity and/or on health promotion' (WHO 2011: 42).

The medicalization of sport was noticeably accelerated by what came to be called the *obesity epidemic*. According to Gard and Wright (2004), discourse about obesity consists of the following beliefs: (i) populations are getting heavier and that average body weight is increasing rapidly; (ii) obesity is a global problem; (iii) obesity is caused by lifestyle factors (such as the excessive use of computers, watching television, etc., which directly lead to a lack of physical activity); (iv) obesity is linked to a decline in self-discipline, traditional family values and parenting skills; and (v) obesity policy should focus particularly on children, because the behaviour of this population can most easily be modified and controlled. Indicatively, the UK Department of Health's *Tackling Obesities: Future Choices* (DoH 2007) estimated that, by 2015, 36% of males and 28% of females in the UK would be obese. Although estimates vary, there is widespread consensus that obesity costs each state billions of pounds each year and that related costs are continually rising. In 2013, obesity ceased to be seen solely as a health risk factor, and became re-defined by the American Medical Association (AMA) as a disease in itself.

While the rhetoric continues, the predicted health crisis has not entirely emerged (UK obesity levels remained below 25% in 2013) and, despite extensive scientific endeavours, the links between obesity and (ill-)health remain uncertain (Gard 2010). The obesity epidemic has therefore entered a new phase signalled by what might be termed a shift from fatness to fitness, as calls have increasingly been made in the medical world to tackle a *global inactivity pandemic* (Piggin and Bairner 2016). Notable amongst such calls was the *Lancet Physical Activity Series* published in July 2012 (Lancet 2012). This collection of empirical articles and commentaries positioned physical activity as 'the fourth leading cause of death worldwide' (Kohl *et al.* 2012: 294), responsible for 6–10% of all 57 million deaths from major non-communicable diseases per year worldwide (Lee *et al.* 2012). Accordingly, an ever-expanding evidence base for the health benefits of regular exercise depicts regular physical activity as significant in reducing an individuals' risk of suffering from breast cancer, colon cancer, diabetes, heart disease, hypertension and stroke. In total, it has been promoted as part of the effective management of over 20 chronic conditions (DoH 2011) including cerebrovascular disease, depression, osteo- and rheumatoid arthritis, osteoporosis and chronic obstructive pulmonary disorder (COPD). More generally, physical activity is thought to contribute to musculoskeletal health, workplace wellness and sustainable living (Jones *et al.* 2011; RCP 2012). Physical inactivity now constitutes one of the 'big four' proximate causes of preventable ill-health, alongside smoking, excessive alcohol intake and poor nutrition (AMRC, 2015).

However, central to distinguishing these trends from what might be termed the healthicization of society (Conrad 1992), is the explicit attempt to claim that 'Exercise is Medicine'. The Exercise is Medicine (EiM) campaign launched in November 2007 as a collaborative initiative of the American College of Sports Medicine (ACSM) and the AMA (Sallis 2009) and is now established in 43 countries (Neville 2013). We discuss EiM in greater detail later in the book (see Chapters 4 and 6) but for now it is sufficient to note that this literal and metaphorical claim to the medicinal qualities of physical activity has been supported by one notable study, which concluded that: 'exercise and many drug interventions are often potentially similar in terms of their mortality benefits in the secondary prevention of coronary heart disease, rehabilitation from stroke, treatment for heart failure, and prevention of diabetes' (Naci and Ioannidis 2013: 1).

Concurrent with the processes defined above, it has become noticeable that sport appears to be increasingly dependent on medicine for its effective functioning. Perhaps most fundamentally, athletes' (in)ability to *participate* is often biomedically determined. For instance, sport participation is frequently preceded by medical assessment of physical function/limitation, most notably in the boundary-blurring case of Oscar Pistorius who sought to run in both the London Olympic and Paralympic Games in 2012. Biomedical science has similarly been invoked to adjudicate upon the cases of Caster Semenya and Dutee Chand. The former was suspended by the International Amateur Athletic Federation (IAAF) for nine months after winning the women's 800 m at the 2009 World Athletics Championship amid media speculation over her sex, while the latter successfully appealed to the Court of Arbitration for Sport (CAS) against her indefinite ban from competition due to the discovery of testosterone levels outside the 'normal' range for a female. Medical personnel similarly make key interventions during sports competitions. A particularly notable case involved the Bolton Wanderers' footballer, Fabrice Muamba, who suffered a heart attack during a live televised game in an English FA Cup match in 2012. Muamba was treated on the pitch for over 70 minutes. He survived, but subsequently retired from professional football due to his underlying heart condition. The incident sparked debates about the role and value of cardiac screening in sport, which will be further explored later in this book (see Chapter 10). The management of concussion has also become a major issue (see Chapter 9), illustrated in the 2014 FIFA World Cup Final when Germany's Christoph Kramer received lengthy treatment for a head injury, but was allowed to carrying on playing for a further 10 minutes. So high a profile has the issue become, that President Obama personally addressed the 'Healthy Kids and Safe Sports Concussion Summit' at the White House in May 2014. Yet, as illustrated by the sacking of Chelsea FC doctor Eva Carneiro in 2015, medical intervention in sport can be fraught with tensions as coaching/managerial staff seek to direct medical matters and question the expertise of healthcare professionals (BBC 2015a; see Chapters 7 and 8).

Concentration on such high profile incidents reveals the exceptional rather than the routine aspects of medical provision for elite athletes for, as Kevin Young (1993: 373) presciently remarked some time ago, 'by any measure, professional sport is a violent and hazardous workplace, replete with its own unique form of "industrial disease"'. Recognition of this periodically re-surfaces in the campaigns of medical associations to ban combat sports, such as boxing and mixed martial arts. Less publicly but no less significantly, those bidding to host sport mega-events are obliged to promise a wealth of medical services and resources. For instance, at the London 2012 Olympic Games three 'polyclinics' were established at the main and two satellite Olympic villages. Medical support was also made available at each of the training and competition venues and, while partly dependent on the injury risk of the respective sports, generally included physiotherapy, sports massage, field of play recovery teams, athlete-dedicated ambulance services, sports medicine physicians and, in some cases, dental services. It was anticipated that a total of 3000 volunteers would be required to provide healthcare support at the games (EMJ 2008). Additionally there were 11 designated Olympic hospitals (LOCOG 2012) with 12 on-call consultants and regularly scheduled clinics (including cardiology, dermatology, neurology and surgery). The British National Health Service (NHS) provided physiotherapy and other musculoskeletal treatments, diagnostic imaging and laboratory tests at the request of national team doctors. In contrast to the normal means-testing system for British citizens, designated pharmacies provided free prescriptions to Olympic athletes. All this was *in addition* to the medical provision that national Olympic committees (NOCs) provided for their own teams and which normally deal with the vast majority of athlete injuries (Junge *et al.* 2009). The United States Olympic Committee (USOC), for instance, brought a reported 85 medical staff to support 530 athletes competing in London (Beaumont 2012).

While such interventions are sometimes predicated on the conventional medical focus of restoring health – for instance, in light of the surge in stories of professional athletes experiencing mental health problems, the English Premier League has made it compulsory for football clubs to appoint a mental health first-aider (Hughes 2014) – a distinct feature of medical practice in sport is the prominence of performance concerns. Sometimes these activities are routine but again, at their extreme, they have led to media controversy and indeed serious ethical questions about the work of healthcare personnel in sport. In particular, juridical cases and journalistic and autobiographical exposés have increasingly raised awareness of the degree to which elite sport is dependent on drug regimes. For example a *Sunday Times* (3 April 2016) investigation secured video evidence of Dr Mark Bonar's claims to have provided illegal performance-enhancing drugs to 150 British elite athletes from sports including professional football, tennis, boxing, cycling and cricket. Bonar had previously been investigated by the UK Anti-Doping Agency (UKAD) which concluded that the privately practising, anti-ageing specialist was beyond their jurisdiction. They referred the case to the General Medical Council (GMC), which took no action and, by the time the media exposé broke, his registration had lapsed. While at the time of writing no legal action had been taken (collusion in performance-enhancement in sport is against GMC regulations but is not illegal under British law) the case bore considerable similarities to the 2013 prosecution of Madrid-based doctor, Eufemiano Fuentes (Malcolm and Smith 2015).

The ethical challenges endemic to sports medicine practice were particularly exposed in the 'Bloodgate' scandal in English rugby union in 2009 (Anderson 2011). The case involved the conspiracy of Harlequins RFC medical staff to: (a) fake a blood injury (thereby enabling a player to be substituted for tactical advantage); and (b) purposefully cut and then stitch the player in order to obscure the previous deception. The incident led the physiotherapist (Stephen Brennan) to be struck off by the Health Professions Council (HPC) after admitting supplying fake blood capsules to players (later repealed), and the club doctor (Wendy Chapman) to be reprimanded by the GMC after admitting intentionally causing a patient harm (she escaped harsher punishment after claiming extenuating circumstances of depression following treatment for cancer).

So fundamental is the medical 'team behind the team' for the everyday functioning of sport that certain facilities and individuals develop celebrity status. Notable in European football is the MilanLab, a 'high tech interdisciplinary scientific research centre' established in 2002 by Italian team AC Milan. The facility has been accredited with prolonging the careers of many Milan players, and has been supported by personal testimonies of celebrity footballers. For instance, treatment following the diagnosis of a dental complaint resolved David Beckham's back problem which had, in turn, impeded his running. Subsequently Beckham was able to resume training and lost half his body fat (Brewin 2011). Within British sport perhaps the most notable healthcare provider of recent years has been Steve Peters. Peters was originally accredited with helping the British cycling team to unprecedented Olympic success in Beijing (2008) and has subsequently worked with Liverpool FC, the England national football team and snooker player Ronnie O'Sullivan. Peters describes himself as a sports psychiatrist (although sports psychologists are rather more prevalent in sport), and is famed for his approach to maximizing performance through enabling athletes to control their 'inner chimp'. In the United States, surgeons such as Frank Jobe and James Andrews have similarly been feted for their contribution to saving the careers of a variety of elite sportspeople. Conversely, Stephen Dank became notorious for the 'supplement programme' he introduced at Essendon FC (an Australian-rules football team). Kept secret from the club doctor, Bruce Reid, the intervention of this sports scientist ultimately led to 34 past and present players being banned for doping offences (Crawford 2016).

Celebrity sports medics epitomize how the medicalization of elite sport impacts upon the broader sports culture; how 'elite sport and the structures that support it, such as sports medicine, are at the forefront of public consciousness' (McEwen and Taylor 2010: 88). For instance, it was as a consequence of an injury to the aforementioned David Beckham prior to the 2002 Football World Cup that metatarsals became cemented in the British *lingua franca* (Carter 2007). Clinicians anecdotally report that media coverage of elite sport influences patients' treatment expectations (Milne 2011), and there was a reported rise in the public demand for sports physiotherapy services following the London 2012 Olympics (Owen 2012). While in the US it is not unusual for a doctor to pay in excess of $1 million for the right to be identified as the appointed physician to a professional sports team (Dunn *et al.* 2007), even in the more commercially limited UK healthcare market, the vibrant and growing private sector exploits links with elite sport. For instance, Dave 'Rooster' Roberts, a physiotherapist contracted to Lancashire County Cricket Club utilizes testimonials from elite athletes and, in particular, his most famous client, Andrew Flintoff, to endorse his private physiotherapy practice. Flintoff says:

His no nonsense approach to diagnosing, treating and rehabilitation numerous injuries over the years helped me get the best out of my body. A number of serious operations meant many hours in rehab but Rooster always gave me the confidence to know that I would recover and I trust his judgment. I know from my experiences, having seen him and his team of physios at close quarters, that no matter who you are you are always given the same high standard of care. Thank you!

Either because it is taken as indicative of quality, or because the primary demand for such services stems from sport injuries, private physiotherapy care is frequently marketed through a 'sport' appendage. Of the 15 'physiotherapy' businesses identified in one UK county (Leicestershire) via a search of the online directory Yell.com, five used the word sport in their title, 11 cited sports injuries in their marketing, and another was physically located at a community rugby club (search conducted 30 March 2016). Notable in the above examples is the commingling of sports medical and para-medical professions in the media and public imagination (a point further developed in Chapters 7 and 8).

The convergence of both elite and mass participation sport, and medicine and health, is particularly well illustrated by the rise of urban marathon running. For instance, the London Marathon combines a race for international-standard athletes who compete for around £150,000 (Abbott World Marathon Majors 2015), with an event open to approximately 38,000 members of the general public. Here, then, elite sport and the exercising public both spatially overlap and, owing to the extensive physical demands, psychologically converge. The public can take part by either entering an open ballot (where approximately one in five applicants is accepted) or by acquiring one of the places guaranteed to charities, the vast majority of which raise money for medically-related causes. These charities attract runners via advertisements premised on a trope of the prevalence and severity of illness in modern society, the achievements of biomedicine and the prospect of more effective future treatment. Concomitantly, these events foreground participants as fundamentally healthy, disciplined and actively seeking self-improvement. Consequently, 'the marathon as a media event and an embodied experience reflects and helps to perpetuate an individualization and medicalization of illness' and thus might be considered 'the most visible contemporary spectacle of health' (Nettleton and Hardey 2006: 457).

Yet contrary to this, and largely hidden from public view, are the health costs of marathon participation. For instance, organizers of the London Marathon advise participants in this 'spectacle of health' that they should only compete with the agreement of their family physician. Additionally, they anticipate that 25% of those who enter (i.e. about 13,000 people) will fail to even start the race due to injury or illness contracted in the lead-up to the event (Symons 2016). For those who do participate, the route is punctuated by more than 40 first aid stations, including cardiac units and resuscitation facilities. There are two 'field hospitals' at the finish line and local 'receiving hospitals' bolster their provision with St John's ambulance volunteers. In total, there are approximately 1000 St John's and 100 physiotherapist volunteers available on the day (Tunstall Pedoe n.d.). Despite this provision, the manifest injury impact of marathon running is significant. There have been 11 deaths in the London Marathon since 1981 (by comparison, over the same period 27 horses have died in the Grand National leading groups such as *Animal Aid* to campaign for the abolition of this 'morally unacceptable' event). A survey following the Canterbury (New Zealand) marathon found that 90% of runners reported developing a specific health problem associated with taking part in the event (Satterthwaite *et al.* 1999). The scale of medical provision for a major urban marathon was vividly described by Dr David Driscoll following the 2013 terrorist attack at the Boston Marathon. Driscoll (2013), head of medical services for the race, described the readiness of his team to deal with the emergency: 'We run it as a MASH [Mobile Army Surgical Hospital] unit and ... it's interesting because we've been told that when we're doing it, it's an organized disaster because of the volume of runners that come through there'. Few other events, ironically, would have been as well resourced to deal with the 264 or more individuals injured in the bomb blast.

We can see therefore that the relationships between sport, medicine and health are wide-ranging. The fusion of medicine and healthcare in elite and mass level sport is indicative of the centrality of this nexus in contemporary society yet a study revealing that charity parachute jumps cost the British NHS £13.75 in healthcare costs for every £1 raised shows the ironic reality of this idealized relationship (Lee *et al.* 1999). In the next two sections we begin to scratch beneath the surface of this relationship by exploring two underpinning ideas, namely that sports participation is a fundamental and necessary part of a healthy lifestyle; and that elite sport rationally exploits science and medicine in the pursuit of competitive success. The chapter concludes by sketching out the broad approach and content of the book.

The sport–health ideology

The link between sport and health – the sport–health ideology – is one of the more enduring human beliefs. Waddington (2000) identifies the historic and cross-cultural ubiquity of these ideas, dating back to Ancient Greek societies, and held with equal vigour in the capitalist and communist, highly developed and developing, nations of the twentieth century. The universality of such ideas alerts us to the fact that throughout most of human history evidence for the connection has been somewhat tenuous. While increasing in volume and validity, evidence for the health-enhancing qualities of exercise that medical science has produced in recent years has not shifted paradigmatically but has, rather, essentially corroborated folk-loric wisdom; moderate rather than extensive physical activity is good for one's heart.

Problematically though, a common characteristic of the sport–health ideology is the conflation of sport and exercise (Waddington 2000) which, in its contemporary iteration, has been extended to embrace physical activity. Traditionally, sport has been defined in terms of organized and institutionally recognized contests which are playful and non-utilitarian, and more physical than intellectual, in character (Guttmann 1978). While rigid adherence to such definitions obscures the multidimensional character of sport, and in particular the sport-like activities of relatively marginalized groups (Malcolm 2012), it does enable us to distinguish sport from related but nonetheless meaningfully distinct activities. Specifically, exercise is less formally structured, not especially playful, more utilitarian (undertaken to improve 'fitness' perhaps), but potentially just as vigorous. Physical activity has come to be used as an all-encompassing term to embrace sport-like and less energetic activities than exercise and to categorize aspects of daily living – e.g. gardening or walking – as health-enhancing forms of movement (see Chapter 4).

However, while public perception and state policies tend to conflate sport, exercise and (now) physical activity, the type of social relations which characterize those activities advocated as health-promoting – moderate, rhythmic and gentle – have very different health outcomes to the organized, competitive physical games that are sports (Waddington 2000). For instance, in recognition of the incidence of injury in elite sport, the International Olympic Committee (IOC) has conducted audits at each Summer and Winter Games since Beijing in 2008. During London 2012, for instance, this revealed an injury rate of 128.8 injuries and 71.7 illnesses per 1000 athletes (Engebretsen et al. 2013). The surveys demonstrate the enormous variation between sports, with nearly 40% of those participating in Taekwondo, 35.2% of footballers and 21.8% of handball players, but just 1.6% of those competing in archery, reporting new or recurring injuries (the research design excluded pre-existing or ongoing injuries). Even this probably under-reports the full extent of the phenomenon, due to the logistical problems of ensuring survey completion across multiple venues/days, and from NOCs with more limited medical staffs (Junge et al. 2009). Indicatively, data reviewing injuries throughout the 2010 International Skiing Federation season suggested that the IOC's findings for the Vancouver (Winter) Games underestimated injury incidence by 31% (Engebretsen et al. 2013).

To put the injury incidence in elite sport into perspective, Hawkins and Fuller (1999) compared government injury data across occupations. They noted that there are an estimated 710 injuries per 100,000 working hours in professional football in the UK, which compares unfavourably with both the national average (0.36 per 100,000 working hours) and traditionally hazardous occupations such as mining and quarrying (1.3 injuries per 100,000 working hours). Ultimately, the occupational injury rates in UK professional football are 2000 times greater than the national average, and 500 times greater than the next most high-risk occupations. While these data identified frequency rather than severity of injury, the extent to which elite sport is more dangerous than all other occupations is just as striking as it is indicative of the ubiquity of the sport–health ideology. It shows the propensity to assess the health-promoting qualities of sport-related activities according to the 'minority of the best' (Elias and Scotson 1994) rather than a holistic analysis of the outcomes of human participation in these activities.

In attempting to explain the high degree of injury-tolerance amongst elite athletes, sociologists of sport have invoked the notion of the 'culture of risk' (Frey 1991). The culture of risk structures (and is structured by) athletes' expectations to normalize the experience of playing with pain and injury. Here, the willingness to sacrifice one's health in order to carry on playing while injured or in pain is viewed as necessary for anyone aspiring to sporting success. Athletes thus find themselves immersed in what Nixon (1992) describes as the 'risk-pain-injury-paradox'; that is to say, a context in which the commitment to achieve sporting success (evident in the propensity to play whilst injured) leads the individual to exacerbate their impairment, ultimately undermining the chances of sporting success. The depth of commitment to this culture of risk, and the degree to which identities are bound to the role of athlete, mean that those who were unable to train/compete experience feelings of self-blame, guilt, depression and uncertainty about their future careers (Roderick et al., 2000). Athletes also speak of their strained relationships with partners and families, and demonstrate a strong desire to return to playing and training as soon as possible after injury. Some sports reward aggressive masculinity and participants who inflict violence on opponents, while prevailing economic relations may have led to the increased health-harming competitiveness of sport, including for instance the more experimental use of performance-enhancing drugs.

Although the level of competition (elite versus mass) intensity and type of sport (contact versus non-contact) significantly shape health outcomes, cultural factors constrain the behaviour of all sport and exercise participants in ways that promote risk-taking and thus incidence of injury. For example, two auto-ethnographic studies highlight how the experiences of elite and non-elite athletes are similar in kind (if not degree). Allen-Collinson's (2005) description of the aftermath of a knee injury sustained while running includes determined attempts to carry on exercising by adapting training routines, extensive investigation of self-help sources, reluctant and unproductive engagements with healthcare professionals and, ultimately, a two-year recovery beset by various re-injury setbacks. Similarly Dashper's (2013) account of sustaining facial injuries in an equestrianism accident not only shows the ubiquity of the culture of risk in sport (e.g. through instinctive attempts to carry on riding), but the equally identity-defining character of participation in non-competitive, leisure-based, sports. Dashper describes how the longer term impact of the injury entailed diminished athletic participation, feelings of vulnerability and the generation of a deep sense of frustration. Consequently, we see that, 'athletic injury remains a part of the self-concept long after the wounds have healed' (Dashper 2013: 335). The ideological link between sport and health is therefore far from straightforward and, while evidence for health benefits relates rather more to exercise than to sport per se, all such activities entail a greater or lesser frequency of participant harm that is fundamental to any assessment of the medicalization of sport. The epidemiology of sport-related injury (SRI) is discussed in detail in Chapter 4, while the exercising public's subjective experiences of injury form the basis of Chapter 5.

Aside from the conflation of activity types, and the related failure to fully recognize the unintended injury consequences of these activities, three further critiques of the sport–health ideology have been made. First, dependence on commercial sponsorship leads elite sport to promote fundamentally unhealthy lifestyles. Criticisms were initially focused on the appropriation of sport by alcohol and tobacco companies (see, for example, Waddington 2000), but due to subsequent legislative changes, concern is now more frequently raised in relation to companies such as McDonalds and Coca-Cola, which use sports mega-events to promote their high calorie, fat- and sugar-rich food and drinks to an international audience, in direct contravention to public health nutrition messages (Mansfield and Malcolm 2014). Second, prevailing economic relations have fostered consumerist ideas that lead exercise participation to increasingly take the form of what might be described as 'cosmetic fitness' (e.g. Scambler *et al.* 2004). Third, the sports–health ideology can be criticized for its propensity to individualize responsibility for health affairs. Safai (2008) notes that this process of individualization leads the 'social determinants of health' (Wilkinson and Marmot 2003) to become obscured, as sport and health promotion policies frequently neglect the barriers that exist for disadvantaged and marginalized populations and invoke victim-blaming (more on this in Chapter 6).

As illuminating as these critiques are, there is scope to develop a more nuanced understanding of the sport–health ideology. First we need to appreciate the dynamic character of sport and health. Both are subject to historical change in ways that fundamentally alter their mutual intersection and respective interdependence with medicine. Not only has the organization of competitive sports changed over the last 25 years (see next section), but the concept of health and its social significance have shifted too (see Chapter 2). Second, we should consider the role of medicine in mediating the sport–health ideology, for it has become evident that (sports) medicine has become increasingly complicit in the reproduction of ideas linking sport and health (see Chapter 3), arguably for its own self-serving ends. Third, we also need to more fully appreciate the degree to which 'sport' goes to protect the sport–health ideology (see Chapters 9 and 10). The ideology is perpetuated by sports administrators who operate in a competitive commercial and public funding environment. Ironically, upholding the sport–health ideology while neglecting the counterfactual evidence may have significant health-harming consequences. Despite these critiques, there appears to be minimal opposition to the sport–health ideology vocalized in contemporary discourses of sport, medicine and health.

Sport and the rational exploitation of science

A second widely accepted, but potentially problematic, idea addressed in this book is that the 'post-Second World War rationalization of sport, marked by an emphasis on performance, has provided an expanding marketplace for medical and health professions to apply their expertise' (Theberge 2009a: 278). However, before exploring the major dynamics of change in twentieth and twenty-first century sport we must briefly account for the ubiquity of sport in contemporary culture.

Sports, in their modern form, have existed since the 1700s. Guttmann's (1978) Weberian-informed account argues that modern sport's seven distinct characteristics – secularism, equality, specialization, bureaucratization, rationalization, quantification and obsession with records – can be linked to Protestantism and the emergence of rational-scientific epistemologies in eighteenth-century Western Europe. While Marxists (e.g. Hargreaves 1986) have linked these developments to the growth of capitalism – notably many sports were first codified or formalized in England where the capitalist mode of production was particularly advanced – Elias (1986a; 1986b) argued that these distinctly rule-bound activities emerged in relation to the development of stricter levels of personal self-control and discipline characteristic of the habitus changes entailed in the European civilizing processes (Elias 2000).

In an extension of these ideas, Elias and Dunning (1986) developed the notion of the quest for excitement. They argued that in these relatively 'safe' and pacified societies people tend to seek those emotions – fear, anxiety, anger, sadness – which they otherwise rarely encounter (or avoid) in 'real life'. A delicate balance between routine (which provides security) and de-routine (which provides playful risk and insecurity) is key. Such 'controlled and enjoyable de-controlling of restraints on emotions' (Elias and Dunning 1986: 65) is enhanced in collective activities (e.g. spectating at organized events or taking part in team sports) for this makes the sport/ leisure experience mutually reinforcing, distinctive and therefore more meaningful. Sport provides this kind of 'excitement' in a way that regular routinized exercise for the pragmatic pursuit of health does not and cannot. In arguing that Elias and Dunning underplayed the degree to which sport and leisure participation involves the quest for self-realization and identity formation, Maguire (1992) suggests that a more accurate conceptualization positions engagement with sport as a quest for exciting significance. People, either personally (as participants) or vicariously (as spectators), pursue 'exciting' *and* identity-generating activities. The characteristics of quantification and rationalization that define *modern* sport mean that, at all levels of participation, meaning is often generated by heightened levels of exertion in the search for new levels of physical attainment.

During the twentieth century, commercialization and politicization became the primary factors shaping (elite) sport into identity-meaningful activities. In *Faster, Higher, Stronger*, Beamish and Ritchie (2006) argue that the rational pursuit of enhanced human athletic performance (and the quest for commercially-rewarded and/or nationally prestigious victory), has led sport to become 'an intensive, exhaustive occupation where athletes are fully embroiled in sophisticated training regimes utilizing scientifically developed technologies that create long-term physiological and personality changes as they progress through the high-stakes, "winner-takes-all" road to the pinnacle of world-class sport' (Beamish and Ritchie 2006: 8). However, the public's media-driven focus on medal winning performances obscures the reality of 'detailed labor whereby underpaid athletes train relentlessly to keep pace with others who are also single-mindedly pursuing their own assault on the limits of human athletic performance' (Beamish and Ritchie 2006: 139). While Beamish and Ritchie focused on the increased use of performance-enhancing substances (itself, as noted above, deeply implicating medicine) they depict the injury and ill-health characteristic of the culture of risk not simply as an unintended consequence, but one of 'a number of deeply embedded occupational hazards and health risks that are integral' to sport (Beamish and Ritchie 2006: 123).

Beamish and Ritchie (2006) essentially extend the thesis of John Hoberman's (1992) seminal historical sociology of sports medicine, *Mortal Engines*. Arguing that contemporary sport can be conceived of as a large if disorganized biological experiment, Hoberman (1992: 19) notes that 'sport and medicine ... developed a symbiotic relationship during the twentieth century'. Initially 'sport served the ends of science' (Hoberman 1992: ix), with athletes simply a source of interesting physiological data. They were, moreover, just one amongst a range of atypical groups – notably manual workers and military personnel – and biomedical scientists deemed them less significant than those whose social contribution included economic production and national defence. However, the overriding rationale for experimentation on all these demographic groups was to learn more about the 'normal' functioning of the human body. In this respect, sports medicine emerged as part of the 'new biological science of man' (Hoberman 1992: 6). It embodied a broader struggle between traditional beliefs in the fixed limit of human biology and modernist conceptions of unlimited (or hitherto unreached) potential. Reflecting these themes, physicians were somewhat divided over whether (vigorous) exercise had detrimental consequences for health (particularly for 'vulnerable' populations including women), or whether such beliefs were both refutable and retarding human progress. They were, though, united in their belief that these physical marvels did not require medical improvement. However, as the development of professional, commercial and international sport placed a greater premium on the value of winning, relations with sports science morphed such that, by the end of the twentieth century, challenges to the sport–health ideology not only dissipated but, more importantly, physiology had 'been put in the service of sport' (Hoberman 1992: 74).

Waddington (1996) usefully connects these sport-related developments with the broader concept of medicalization. His analysis of the development of sports medicine literature illustrates how athletes have become defined as a distinct population whose need for continuous medical support is akin to the needs of the chronically ill; the widespread acceptance of the idea that, 'athletes require routine medical supervision, not because they necessarily have a clearly defined pathology but ... simply because they are athletes' (Waddington 1996: 197). Athletes, moreover, have not simply welcomed these developments but have actively sought to increase their access to medical interventions in the search for competitive success. For Waddington, the conjuncture of these two relatively autonomous processes accounts for the contemporary manifestation of sports medicine in which performance-enhancement has 'become an important part of the *raison d'être*' (Waddington 1996: 185).

While accounts of the rational application of medical science in sport are important, the thesis is limited by the centrality of performance-enhancing/illicit drug use. Consequently, these theories are disconnected from, and unable to account for either the institutional manifestation, or the 'everyday' practice, of sports medicine. The former appears to have been a somewhat laborious process (see Chapter 3) while the latter is often manifest in relatively ad-hoc forms (see Chapters 7–9). A further unintended consequence of the focus on this 'obsessional and often corrupt subculture' (Hoberman 1992: x) is the homogenization of sports medicine and thus the tendency to underplay conflicts within the 'professional project' of sports medicine, or between sports medicine and the wider profession. Finally, it portrays sports medicine as almost entirely devoid of agency, developing along a singular logic rather than in polymorphous ways. As Heggie (2011: 6) notes, 'considering sports medicine as a multi-faceted practice adds depth and context' to our understanding. Recognition of this alerts us to the benefits of a sustained engagement with the sociology of medicine/health and illness.

Towards a sociology of sport, medicine and health

Despite the visibility of multiple and complex interconnections between sport, medicine and health, a review of the literature shows that there has been a notable lack of interest in these phenomena outside the sociology of sport (Malcolm and Safai 2012). In part this might be explained in relation to the way the parameters of the sociology of medicine/health and illness have developed and been defined. Initially termed 'medical sociology', concerns emerged that the field was overly oriented towards producing research that enhanced the efficiency of medicine (e.g. alleviating patient management issues). Preference for the term 'sociology of medicine' signalled a more critical questioning of the role and functioning of medicine itself and thereby located the subdiscipline more directly within the sociological studies per se. Finally, the move to a 'sociology of health and illness' is: (a) a product of understanding that medicine is not some kind of benign body that responds to human problems, but is fundamental to the social development of health and illness; (b) a recognition that the social significance of health and illness expands far beyond patients' interface with medicine; and (c) a belief in the importance of serving the interests of people who experience illness and ill-health. The relatively late formalization of a medical subspeciality (sports medicine) to 'serve', its ambiguous role regarding the development of performance relative to the promotion of health, and a belief that patient suffering is probably less extreme than in other areas of medicine – augmented, of course, by the ubiquity of the sport–health ideology – may have inhibited the exploration of the sport-medicine-health nexus. But, as this book demonstrates, the sociology of medicine/health and illness is enhanced by an understanding of the various and multifaceted role of sport/exercise/physical activity in contemporary medicine and health. A holistic analysis of health and illness can no longer ignore these important areas of medical practice.

Conversely, and while it is recognized that a number of existing studies of sport have applied key concepts from the sociology of medicine/health and illness (notably Roderick 2006; Sparkes and Smith 2002; Theberge 2008; Thing 2012; Waddington and Murphy 1992), a more rigorous engagement with the perspectives and knowledge generated in the sociology of medicine/health and illness will significantly enhance the sociology of sport. The sociology of health and illness broadly consists of: the analysis of medical knowledge; lay perceptions and experiences of health and illness; social and cultural aspects of the body; the patterned nature of health and illness in relation to the wider social structure, and the social organization of formal and informal health care (Nettleton 2006). Turner (1995) similarly argues that a comprehensive analysis should embrace three levels: the *individual*, or perceptions of healthcare; the *social*, or the construction of disease categories and healthcare organizations; and the *societal*, or healthcare systems in their political context. More recently Timmermans (2013) has argued that the unique contribution of what he calls qualitative health sociology can be seen in seven distinct 'warrants': exploring the social construction of beliefs; reframing dominant perspectives; charting the winners and losers of health interventions; identifying the unfulfilled promises of medicine; exploring the experiences of medicine and health across multiple contexts; exposing the impact of economic interests; and revealing how social relations mediate the impact of medical and health interventions. The contents of this book resonate with the spectrum of concerns identified in each of these broad typologies

In the following chapters the relationships between sport, medicine and health are explored in four heuristically discrete, but in reality interacting, stages. An underlying rationale for the order is to move from the general to the more specific but, in saying that, it should be noted that one of the fundamental merits of the scale of this project and its primary focus on a particular branch/field/subspeciality of medicine, is the ability to analyse human behaviour in the round, to identify the interdependence of the structural level of social change with the micro-level analysis of (illness) experience and interactions (Elias 1978). Thus, the next two chapters provide foundational work, setting out the conceptual and theoretical framework for the analysis and developmentally examining institutional aspects of the medicalization of sport to illustrate its core concerns and constituencies, its successful and stilted initiatives. The primary focus of Chapters 4–6 is the impact of the medicalization of sport on the public, starting with an exploration of the most visible and socially pervasive manifestation of the sport-health-medicine nexus (Physical Activity Health Promotion (PAHP)), examining the social construction of beliefs that largely operate at the societal or conceptual level. Moreover, using evidence of lay perceptions and experiences of the health and illness related to sport/exercise/physical activity these chapters contrast the success of such policies in establishing social awareness with their relative failure on the interactional level. In this regard, the chapters speak most directly to the sport–health ideology discussed above. The third stage (Chapters 7–8) switches empirical focus to elite sport, including the social processes that determine healthcare provision and socially construct conceptualizations of illness as part of the social and cultural formation of the athletic body. It reveals the intersection of dominant perspectives, economic interests and the unfulfilled promise of medicine (relative, especially, to para-medical professions). In this regard, it speaks most directly to notions of the rational exploitation of medical science in the pursuit of athletic performance. In the fourth and final stage we focus on two empirical issues – concussion injuries and cardiac screening – which return us to a more integrated analysis of elite and mass sports medicine and health and of the conceptual, institutional and interactional levels of medicalization. In contrast to the somewhat limited integration evidenced in Chapters 7 and 8, we see medicine more proactively and successfully taking an interventionist role, but one that is fundamentally underpinned by the sport–health ideology and its relative importance to the functioning and economic viability of elite sport. In the final chapter we directly assess the medicalization of sport and substantiate the book's central thesis; namely that while sport has been fundamentally shaped by increasing medicalization during the twentieth and twenty-first centuries, the development of medical influence (and jurisdictional control) has been constrained by a combination of the relative autonomy of (elite) sport organizations and personnel, considerations of cost control and limited efficacy, especially as evaluated by lay/patient consumers. Accordingly, medicalization is considerably more 'complete' at the conceptual level, where issues come to be understood in medical terms or through a medical perspective, than it is at the institutional or interactional levels; that is to say, in relation to the actions of sports medicine personnel and/or when dealing with 'patients'. In relation to sport, medicalization is stronger in relation to issue definition than it is in relation to effective implementation (Conrad 2007).

Chapter 2

Medicine, health and sport

Processes and principles

As the examples in the previous chapter illustrate, sport and medicine are ubiquitous contemporary social institutions. Moreover, there are few concepts or ideas quite as widely resonant as that of health. However, breadth of use often detracts from analytical precision and where the intersections of sport, medicine and health have previously been explored, the complexity and dynamism of each has not always been clearly delineated. While in the previous chapter we outlined some of the core ideas and developments in relation to sport, the aim of this chapter is to explore medicine and health in more detail, to highlight their developmental trajectories and, ultimately, to develop the conceptual framework that enables us to explain their interdependence with sport.

Medicine

Medicine 'originated as a response to human suffering' and such relief 'remains one of the central, defining goals of medicine' (Edwards and McNamee 2006: 104). But in many respects medicine, as alluded to in the sports-related examples discussed, has evolved to be much more than this. To more fully understand the role of medicine in contemporary societies we need to move beyond its definitional properties and look at the contemporary manifestations of this social institution. What are the roots of medicine's social influence, what changes have enabled both the quantitative and qualitative expansion of medicine's scope of practice, and what developments have constrained or challenged medicine as it has become more powerful?

The development of medical power

While medicine's origins are frequently traced back to the Ancient Greeks, a key marker in its modern development is the establishment of the medical *profession*. A profession is a 'special kind of occupation' that has gained control over its own work and become 'autonomous and self directing', able to manage 'clients and problems in its own way' (Freidson 1970: xvii). Professions are able to do this because they are seen to be 'extraordinarily trustworthy', and because they come to be seen as 'authoritative and definitive' in their particular field. According to what became known as the 'trait approach' (MacDonald 1995), any occupation acquiring these characteristics is identified as a profession. However, the basis of medicine's privileged position in contemporary societies is its identification as 'one of the most powerful classic professions' (Saks 1995: 7).

The medical profession's authority rests in part on scientific discovery and technical competence, but also on an organizational coherence, which enables its proponents to convince others that the practice is 'so esoteric or complex that nonmembers of the profession cannot perform the work safely or satisfactorily and cannot even evaluate the work properly' (Freidson 1970: 45). Thus, key markers – or traits – of a profession are the establishment of national organizations (the British Medical Association (BMA) and American Medical Association (AMA) were founded in 1832 and 1847 respectively), and the publication of journals to disseminate specialist knowledge (the *British Medical Journal* and *Journal of the American Medical Association* were founded in 1857 and 1883). Where professions can convince the state of their trustworthy and authoritative status, licence and mandate may be granted (Dingwall 1983). Licence enables a profession to control its own membership. For instance, in the UK the 1858 Medical Act established the GMC which, ever since, has overseen the programme of training which leads to the conferment of the legal status to practice (Larkin 1983). Mandate enables professions to stop others from directly competing in the specified areas of practice. The most successful professions have been able to evaluate and stratify competing types of knowledge (e.g. homeopathy, witchcraft) and occupations (e.g. nursing, physiotherapy) 'so as to limit what they could do and to supervise or direct their activities' (Freidson 1970: 47).

However, critics argue that these characteristics are as much a consequence as they are a cause of professional status. Rather, the existence and persistence of professions can be explained using a variety of alternative perspectives. Freidson's (1970) symbolic interactionist approach placed greatest emphasis on the 'everyday work settings' and the interpersonal relations through which practice and status is negotiated. Doctors therefore are 'more their present than their past ... more an outcome of the pressure of the situation than of what they have earlier "internalized"' (Freidson 1970: 90). Logically, therefore, it matters less what physicians 'know' and 'do' than how their subjects evaluate their knowledge and efficacy. Johnson's (1972) Marxist account locates the development of professions within capitalist state formation, focusing on the producer–consumer relationship and, in particular, on who defines the needs of the consumer and the manner in which those needs are served. Larson's (1977)

Weberian-informed perspective eschews economic determinism to give greater explanatory power to the way occupational groups embark on 'professional projects' to control prevalent ideas about their work, while Abbott (1988: 2) conceptualized an interacting system in which occupational groups' disputes over respective jurisdictions are 'the real, the determining history of the professions'.

The nature of the power of the medical profession has, of course, altered over time. Central to this has been the changing locations in which medicine is performed – from bedside to hospital to surveillance medicine – and the impact of this on practice (Armstrong 1995). Bedside medicine occurred in people's homes with diagnosis derived from the patient (the reported and visually-assessed symptoms). In the late nineteenth/early twentieth centuries, hospital medicine became the dominant model, signalling both a spatial move for treatment to a purpose-built work facility, and a shift in the basis of diagnosis as clinical examination firstly supplemented and latterly superseded patients' reporting of symptoms. Physicians' clinical examinations developed to explore underlying pathological causes to patient-experienced symptoms (Bury 2001). Augmented by laboratory testing, medical knowledge and decision-making become increasingly abstracted from the patient. Pseudonyms for hospital medicine include Western, clinical, pathological or bio medicine.

The subsequent development of surveillance medicine shifts the social space of practice from the hospital to the wider community. Initial manifestations included the early twentieth century medical observations of schoolchildren and prospective military recruits, but the broader emphasis on preventative medicine has led to the examination or screening of a range of asymptomatic populations. Here, medicine clearly goes beyond the rather more limited goal of the relief of suffering. Prevention shifts medicine's focus away from the hospitalized patient's body to the environmental and social context. Correlatively, medical interventions expand into social structure (i.e. identifying which populations suffer ill-health) and agency (i.e. the role of lifestyle). Moreover, health screening necessarily identifies a greater prevalence of 'illness' in the population than self-reported measures ever could because it constitutes a fundamentally different kind of experiment or data gathering. Surveillance medicine leads the distinction between health and illness to become increasingly blurred (Armstrong 1995).

In similar vein, Aronowitz (2009: 425) identified the converged experience of risk and disease as surveillance medicine leads to the identification of disease precursors on a 'continuum of abnormalities'. 'Diagnosis creep' entails identifying and treating pre-disease states. The experience of being at risk of developing a disease becomes indistinguishable from the illness experience of symptomatic patients for whom medical intervention has become largely about disease management rather than treatment. Finally, the 'at-risk' population continually expands as diagnostic thresholds (e.g. for diagnosing diabetes, hypertension or obesity) are revised downwards and structural rewards incentivize clinicians to identify marginal cases (Kreiner and Hunt 2013). With ever-growing numbers receiving medical treatment the ability to self-manage increasingly comes to distinguish the ill from the healthy (Timmermans 2013).

Medicalization

The move towards surveillance medicine entails (further) medicalization; the process whereby, 'more and more of everyday life has come under medical domain, influence and supervision' (Zola 1983: 295). Medicalization was initially a term used to refer to the expansion of medical authority through the definition of certain deviant practices as medically classifiable, and medicine's jurisdictional monopoly over their treatment (Zola 1972). Latterly, medicalization was evoked to describe the embrace of a range of natural aspects of the life-course (e.g. childbirth and ageing) into the domain of medical practice. One corollary of medicalization, therefore, is the expansion of medical subdisciplines, such as paediatric and geriatric medicine. As Waddington (1996) argues, sports medicine has to be considered in this light. In relation to sports medicine, medicalization occurs both through the social control of deviance (i.e. the treatment of sports injury) and the structuring of 'natural' life-course events (i.e. physical inactivity and/or weight gain).

Initial analyses of medicalization not only questioned the legitimacy of the medical profession's expansion, but critiqued the development of medicine as a tool of social control. Medicine's expansion leads non-medical personnel to become de-skilled and thus stripped of the ability to look after themselves. Illich (1975) further argued that medicalization meant that the profession not only cured illness and relieved suffering, but created iatrogenesis, or medically caused or exacerbated illness or social problems. But the depiction of medicalization as intentional and imperialistic floundered as it became clear that the ability and intent of medicine to achieve such goals were easily exaggerated. For instance De Swaan (1989) argued that being called upon to adjudicate on social conflicts (in our case, fitness to play sport) created problems for medicine as taking sides in such political debates threatened to undermine the sense of professional collectivism that contributes to medicine's social power. Thus, 'the profession in its entirety has often been hesitant to expand its empire when opportunity seemed to beckon' (de Swaan 1989: 1168).

Over time medicalization continued but shifted in form as the 'engines of medicalization' proliferated and doctors moved from drivers to 'gatekeepers' of the process (Conrad 2007: 142). Consequently medicalization came to be understood as potentially evident on the conceptual, institutional and interactional levels (Conrad 1992). These levels are evident, respectively, when: biomedical vocabularies come to structure public understanding of particular aspects of social life; when biomedical practices are used to administer social problems; and when biomedical actors become more central to the 'cure' of social problems (Halfmann 2011). We should also be cognisant of the relative willingness of groups to embrace medicalization and their abilities to resist. Considered in this multidimensional way, medicalization can vary from partial to extensive, and can occur either with or without the medical profession, as intentional human action or not. Different branches of medicine are differentially equipped to 'achieve' medicalization.

Decoupling medicalization from medicine may detract from considerations of jurisdictional legitimacy (Davis 2006), but it enables a broader understanding of medicine's changing social role. This conceptualization of medicalization has three advantages. First, it extracts an implicit value judgement from the analysis. Medicalization may entail the expansion of medicine's sphere of influence, but this can be disempowering for medicine and/or highly beneficial to those who experience the process. For instance, people whose condition is formally recognized by medicine are able to more legitimately adopt the Parsonian (1975) 'sick role', with all its incumbent rights (and duties). Second, it enables us to focus on medicalization as a process, in which no one group or institution operates a power monopoly and various parties are highly interdependent (Elias 1978). Third it draws our attention to the possibility and importance of both *de*medicalization (when a 'problem' ceases to be defined in medical terms) and non-medicalization (where aspects of health/illness lay beyond the medical domain). Central here is the possibility that medicalization may not be a simple linear process. For example, as we will see, the medicalization of exercise and physical activity may entail reconceptualization of 'ordinary' aspects of social life in essentially medicinal terms, but concurrently may also lead to the decentring of biomedical actors by members of the 'fitness' industry. The medicalization of elite sport performance has arguably had a greater impact on para-medical professions than on medicine itself (see Chapters 7 and 8).

Thus, counter to the inexorable development of medical authority implied in some of the original analyses, it has been argued (Kelleher *et al.* 1994) that the power of the medical profession has been weakened through *de-professionalization* (the fragmentation of the medical profession, greater degrees of administrative control, and jurisdictional contestation by members of other healthcare professions) and *proletarianization* (changing work conditions, including de-skilling through an extended division of labour). McKinlay and Marceau (2002) identify seven processes that have led to the 'decline of the golden age of doctoring': the state's increasingly equivocal support for medicine; the bureaucratization of medicine evident in the growth of managerial monitoring of medical practice and outcomes; the emergence of a global information age which facilitates access to, and thus partly democratizes, knowledge; the increasing influence of para-medical professions; the shift in medical work from treatment to manage-ment as the control of communicable diseases leads to the prominence of chronic illness and an ageing population; patients' declining deference towards and trust in doctors; the fragmentation of medicine and, at times, oversupply of labour. Sports medicine holds an ambiguous position in rela-tion to these processes, it is historically multidisciplinary, receiving limited and/or only recent state support (Heggie 2011), but is also necessarily linked to the division of medicine into specialisms and thus subject to intra-professional, interprofessional and essentially internal, interpersonal conflicts (Malcolm and Scott 2011). These issues are explored in sub-sequent chapters but for present purposes we focus on two challenges to medicine which are of particular relevance here: the changing nature of medicine's relations with patients, and the changing nature of relations *between* medical providers.

Challenges to medical dominance

Challenges to medical dominance are deeply intertwined with the neoliberal ideologies that dominate healthcare policy in the twenty-first century. Neo-liberalism is underpinned by rationalities that reconceptualize social prob-lems in economic terms. Neoliberalism constructs the individual as rational, active and responsible. In shifting the onus of governance from the state to the individual, health becomes an issue of personal responsibility through the self-management of lifestyle risks. Simultaneously, neoliberalism seeks the delivery of 'lean healthcare' (Waring and Bishop 2010) which entails an emphasis on efficiency, the ascendancy of managerialism over professional-ism and enhanced customer/patient satisfaction through service user involve-ment and shared decision making (Horrocks and Johnson 2014). The shift from paternalism to consumerism in contemporary medical consultations entails a greater emphasis on the exchange of information between doctor and patient, a higher degree of negotiation, a desire to establish mutuality and reciprocity and the increasing importance of 'patient choice'. Barriers to this equalization of power in medical care include questions over: (a) how much control patients wish to have (paradoxically studies show that patients both want to be active agents in healthcare decisions, but also guided by the expertise of their doctors (Lupton 1997)); (b) how easily medical authority can be ceded; and (c) whether such policies increase or exacerbate health inequalities due to the differential abilities of patients to exploit this more democratic configuration.

Fundamental to this process are the challenges posed to medical exper-tise. As hospital medicine became increasingly effective in treating and curing infectious disease, so the social burden of chronic illness increased (in both absolute and relative terms). The greater emphasis on illness management that this necessarily entailed served to revitalize primary care (predominant, for example, in bedside medicine) as both more cost- and medically-effective provision. In so doing, the limited efficacy of biomedicine (evident in both epistemological and clinical uncertainty, and discussed further in Chapter 9) became more exposed and, correlatively, it enabled the subjective patient voice to become increasingly audible (Bury 2001). Lay medical knowledge is primarily derived from the phenomenological experience of illness (hence concepts such as biographical disruption and illness narratives emerged, see Chapters 5 and 6 respectively), and the dissemination or democratization of biomedical information (enhanced in a digital age). Although the relative value or impact of lay and medical knowledge varies (Prior 2003), and lay knowledge tends to pose 'little if any direct challenge to the power of the medical profession' where it is 'disorganised and ad-hoc' (Williams and Popay 1994: 118), lay medical knowledge is very significant in the treatment of sport-related injury (see Chapter 5) and thus remains an essential consideration of the contemporary landscape of sports medicine practice. Studies suggest that elite sport provides a context in which patient-athletes are particularly empowered relative to healthcare professionals (see Chapter 8).

Neoliberal, patient-centred philosophies are also invoked in the move towards healthcare delivery by multidisciplinary teams (MDTs). MDTs are seen to reduce the inefficiencies of professional boundary maintenance while also enhancing expertise through specialization. Consequently, 'the ability to work in [this environment] is deemed a crucial characteristic of the modern health professional' (Martin and Finn 2011: 1051). However, these moves are of particular sociological interest in that the re-consideration of professional jurisdictions that the development of MDTs has entailed can lead to conflict as competing professions seek to challenge or reproduce traditional inter-professional relations (Sanders and Harrison 2008). As will be seen in Chapter 8 sports medicine is frequently delivered by MDTs and aspects of conflict and cooperation shape provision and practice.

Concomitant with the growing influence of MDTs is the growth of complementary and alternative medicines (CAMs). Where a treatment is deemed to be 'complementary' it sits alongside and works with biomedicine (e.g. the use of aromatherapy to relieve pain), but where it is deemed to be 'alternative' (often claimed to be 'holistic') it poses a more fundamental challenge to the philosophy of, and could potentially replace, biomedicine. For example, many CAM advocates reject biomedicine's identification of randomized control trials (RCTs) as the 'gold standard' of knowledge production, and instead emphasize the social and emotional aspects of illness by hyphenating 'dis-ease' (Gale 2011). However, because state recognition and thus public funding for CAMs is limited (in the UK at least), access tends to be contoured by economic class and cultural capital. Uptake is also particularly gendered (Brenton and Elliott 2014). The reasons cited for the increasing popularity of CAMs address recurrent themes: reduced confidence or disenchantment with biomedicine resulting from perceptions of impersonal and/or disempowering practice; questions of efficacy, particularly in relation to biomedicine's ability to treat the rising number of chronic illnesses; the democratization of information that facilitates the exchange of medical and lay knowledge; the perception that CAMs offer less invasive and safer treatment than biomedicine; and resistance to biomedicine's apparent reliance on pharmacology (Baarts and Pederson 2009). Incontrovertibly the development of CAMs is part of a 'new medical pluralism' (Cant and Sharma 1999) which contributes to the de-professionalization and proletarianization of medicine described above. Paradoxically it may entail the de-centring of medical personnel yet the location of a wider range of conditions within an essentially medical paradigm.

Thus, an analysis of the development of sports medicine needs to encompass facilitating processes such as professionalization, as well as the countervailing forces that have restricted medicalization. However, as we will see in the next section, while the influence of the medical profession and individual agents has encountered growing resistance in recent years, the broader development of biomedical discourses to explain aspects of social life (and sport, exercise and physical activity in particular), seems to have advanced relatively unfettered. Inherently tied to these changes has been the reconceptualization of 'health' in contemporary Western societies. It is to this that we now turn.

Health

Fundamental to the development of surveillance medicine is the reconstruction of the distinction between illness and health through the development and changing focus of public health interventions. Pre-enlightenment beliefs that illness was subject to 'God's Will', and early state interventions such as quarantine, gradually gave way to more rational, systematic and modernist programmes (Naidoo and Wills 1994). The British public health movement started (c.1840s) as a response to the health implications of urbanization and industrialization and largely focused on disease prevention (e.g. through improved sanitation and immunization programmes). However between the 1920s and 1970s public health became increasingly related to health education. The Central Council for Health Education was established in 1927 effectively to disseminate information and was thus characterized by a greater emphasis on the role of personal behaviour (i.e. what the individual could do to stop the spread of diseases). From the 1940s, focus shifted again to 'health promotion', underpinned by a belief that changes in daily living not only had immediate benefits for disease prevention, but significant broader health benefits. A contemporary iteration, the New Public

Health (NPH), emerged in the late 1980s and sought a holistic approach to health (promotion), embracing statutory and voluntary organizations, examining the health implications of *all* aspects of public policy and frequently addressing entire populations. It is overseen in the UK today by Public Health England (PHE). NPH was stimulated by four key developments: the diminishing returns of investments in technology; the changing disease burden from infection to chronic non-communicable diseases; the ageing population; and financial pressures on health services (Nettleton 2006).

In charting these developments it is important not to overstate the rational application of medicine. For instance, as Jutel and Buetow (2007) note, notions of health have always been influenced by perceptions of physical appearance. The historical association of beauty, health and moral goodness (and their obverse states: ugliness; ill-health; immorality) continue to 'distort' clinical evaluations of patients. For instance, physicians' perceptions of obese patients as lazy and non-compliant, replicates visually-based 'fatist' prejudice (Murray 2008). Similarly Goudsblom's (1986) developmental analysis of public health concerns identified three enduring trends: the link between ill-health and lack of cleanliness, attempts to ostracize the victims of illness, and the ability of the socially advantaged to distance themselves from the unhealthy/disadvantaged and so avoid 'social pollution'. Thus, while humans depict many aspects of their health-related behaviour as logical extrapolations of scientific and experiential knowledge about disease, such beliefs are invariably ex-post facto rationalizations driven by changes to social and personality structures.

In many respects, concomitant with the development of surveillance medicine, the cultural meaning of health has changed. Robert Crawford's (1980) 'Healthism and the medicalization of everyday life' argued that, in line with the protestant work ethic, contemporary Western populations largely believe that health is something that can and *must* be individually achieved. Accordingly, health has become incorporated into contemporary notions of character, identity and citizenship. Conversely, those who fail to adopt healthy practices are deemed irresponsible, weak and personally culpable. Crawford relates the healthism ideology to feelings of greater personal security and general well-being, the mastery of emotions and self-control, and elements of (moralistic) victim-blaming, all of which serve to stratify populations. He further details the structural factors that shape contemporary healthism, including the fusing of the personal and the political; an antipathetic puritanism in response to the hedonism of the 1960s; the intensification of inter-class status rivalries; and the aforementioned rise of neoliberalism. In subsequent work Crawford (2006) argues that health consciousness has become increasingly unavoidable due, amongst other things, to technological advances, the growth of medical and epidemiological research, greater media coverage of health issues and the expansion of the health product market.

A prominent text within this genre is Deborah Lupton's, *The Imperative of Health* (1995). In a Foucauldian-informed revision of Crawford's work, Lupton argues that social relations are created through public health discourse, that biomedicine is 'a symbolic system of beliefs and a site for the reproduction of power relations, the construction of subjectivity and of human embodiment' (Lupton 1995: 4). Through the imperative of health, citizens come to voluntarily compel themselves to live 'healthily', constructing and normalizing a subject who is 'autonomous, directed at self-improvement, self-regulated, desirous of self-knowledge, a subject who is seeking happiness and healthiness' (Lupton 1995: 11). Furthermore, drawing on Elias' (2000) work on civilizing processes, Lupton suggests that these processes feed upon the social value of the 'civilized body' in contemporary societies. The characteristics of the 'civilized body' are that it is strongly demarcated from its social and natural environment (showing greater sensitivity towards nudity, smells, physical contact, and even the visual manifestations of 'ill-health' such as obesity), is able to rationalize and exert a high degree of control over its emotions, monitors the behaviour of others, and internalizes a demarcated set of rules about appropriate/desirable behaviour and form (Shilling 1993).

Building on the deconstruction of the binary categories of health and illness invoked through surveillance medicine (Armstrong 1995), each individual's health-status comes to be located on a continuum. Health can therefore *only* be assessed relative to the health of others. Illness moves from an embodied present to the management of a potential future risk. Because health and illness can logically coexist (e.g. elite athletes continually participate when injured and at times with underlying pathologies), *every* individual has the potential to become healthier. '[I]ndividualizing health protection, however, has encouraged the growth of self-preoccupation and even obsession with personal well-being'; creating the 'me' generation, 'introspective, selfish and lacking communal consciousness' (Porter 1999: 296). Yet counter to medicalization conceived as imperialism, surveillance medicine locates the 'solution' not solely in medical intervention but increasingly in behavioural manipulation of the population in terms, for instance, of exercise and physical activity. As Porter (1999: 290) notes, 'the new era of missionary health evangelism … owes more … to the long traditions of personal health cultures and the methods of clinical prevention than to state medicine'. For these reasons a key segue between (medicine and) health and sport is the notion of 'fitness'.

Fitness

The relationship between sport and health promotion roughly traces the pattern outlined at the beginning of the previous section. The origins of sport, like medicine, are normally traced back to Ancient Greek civilization and notable Greek physicians espoused a variant of the current EiM message (Berryman 2010). While modern medicine would come to have a somewhat ambivalent relationship with sport (see Chapter 3), the public schools of Victorian Britain, infused with beliefs about social Darwinism and eugenics, forged a close connection with nineteenth-century health movements. Sport was seen to inculcate the mental and physical qualities required to run the planet's largest Empire. Administrative bodies such as the National Playing Fields Association (formed in 1925), like the *health education* movement of the early twentieth century, were largely oriented towards the greater provision of opportunities for people to participate in health-enhancing behaviours (see Carter 2012a). The sport–health ideology even influenced the development of the healthcare professions, playing a prominent role in the establishment of physiotherapy, with the Chartered Society of Massage and Medical Gymnastics, forerunner to the Chartered Society of Physiotherapy (CSP), established in 1920 (Larkin 1983). The subsequent phase of *health promotion* was evident in the emergence of what has been called the 'fitness boom' in the 1970s, epitomized by the emergence of practices such as jogging and aerobics. Contemporary iterations of PAHP policies are essentially manifestations of the NPH. Consistent with Goudsblom's (1986) analysis of the public health interventions across history, the advocacy of physical activity for health predates scientifically reliable supporting evidence (by millennia) and thus needs to be considered in light of broader social processes of knowledge production.

Throughout these periods a belief in the causal relationship between fitness and health – the sport–health ideology – remained strong. While Victorians subscribed to the maxim 'mens sana in corpore sana' (a healthy mind in a healthy body), fashion, moral virtuosity, youthfulness, glamour and the desire to be seen as sexually attractive have become central reasons for exercise participation in contemporary societies (Lupton 1995). Crossley's (2006) ethnography suggests that the primary motive for people to start (though notably not continue) attending a gym is the perceived need to lose weight *and* get fit, which itself is stimulated by threats to the agent's embodied self (the moral significance of weight gain, medical advice about health risks, or a 'scare' signalling a potentially undesirable or disrupted future). But while the aesthetic connotations of fitness overlap with traditional notions equating health and physical appearance (Jutel and Buetow 2007), contemporary conceptions of fitness are historically specific. Like ideologies of health, this paradigm stems from individualization, commercialization and democratization and has acquired a distinct moral imperative (Sassatelli 2000). Although systematic exercise 'acts as a marker of an individual's capacity for self-regulation' (Lupton, 1995: 143), it is also fundamentally shaped in relation to the lived experience, and in particular the increasingly sedentary lives, of the majority of those who live in the West (Smith-Maguire

2008). The 'fit' only acquire distinction in societies in which lack of fitness, believed to be evident through 'fatness', is the norm.

Such is their convergence that health and fitness have become conjoined if not synonymous terms (Glassner 1990). Starting around the 1970s, 'gyms' became 'health and fitness clubs' became simply 'health clubs' (Smith-Maguire 2008). A dedicated media sector emerged promoting active lifestyles and endorsing the exercise proscriptions of medical associations. Alternative body altering techniques (e.g. surgery) appear to lack the authenticity of exercise, and suspicions of vanity are dispelled by the inherent effort of 'working out' (Sassatelli 2000). While in the past exercise and fitness may have been seen as the means to the higher goal of health, Neville (2012: 479) argues that this hierarchy has been reversed such that, 'it is now commonly thought that fitness is the most desirable state of the individual's body in modern society – something akin to the new health'. In this respect, 'The health field has contributed medical legitimacy and political currency to participation in physical activity and exercise' (Smith-Maguire 2008: 50). It should be noted, however, that a fundamental aspect of the power of the paradigm equating exercise and medicine is the representation of the former as a 'natural' alternative to the apparent limitations of contemporary biomedicine. For this reason it displays many of the characteristics of broader challenges to the dominance of medicine exemplified, for example, by the CAM movement, yet within an essentially medical explanatory framework.

Despite the re-invigorated modern manifestation of this enduring interrelationship, there are inherent contradictions in this particular iteration of the sport-medicine-health nexus. As fitness has become reified into an obtainable state, its fundamentally relational character becomes obscured. Fitness, rather, should be conceived in the sense of being able to do something; the 'relationship between a person's psychomotor capacities and the sociomaterial context' (Freund and Martin 2004: 274). Second, fitness has become commodified. Contemporary obsessions about the body mean that an activity which, 'in reality requires little equipment, technical knowledge or specialised space, becomes a complex, expensive and arcane enterprise' (Freund and Martin 2004: 280). Fitness is monopolized by an industry that makes exercise a temporally and spatially discrete rather than socially embedded activity. Not only, therefore, do people become de-skilled and thus positioned as unable to self-manage, but fitness essentially reproduces the class-based contours of health as the opportunities for its realization are structured by material means. Finally, like health (cf. Crawford 2006), fitness creates rather than alleviates anxiety. The reification of health and fitness constructs their essentially elusive character; 'a never-to-be-reached horizon looming forever in the future' (Bauman 2000: 23). Contributing to this is the rather equivocal evidence that exercise is an effective weight loss strategy

(Mansfield and Rich 2013), and the sometimes paradoxical relationship between bodily appearance and the objective and subjective perceptions of health, epitomized for instance, by the pharmaceutical dependence of bodybuilders (Monaghan 2001). Despite these contradictions, 'the idea of a fit body, useful to subjects in their daily lives and an immediate signal of self-control and adaptability, seems to have replaced the modest fatalistic hopes of health' (Sassatelli 2000: 408).

With ironic circularity, the developments of medicine which have contributed to the reconceptualization of health and subsequently fitness enable workers in the exercise industry to engage in professional boundary work. Specifically, the power of the appearance-health-moral virtue connection (disciplined, strong-willed, hardworking) provides fitness trainers with considerable physical capital which, in turn, empowers them to encroach into the traditional domains of the healthcare professions. For example, Hutson (2013) illustrates how both clients and trainers perceived exercise as a form of health work. The activities of trainers overlap with those of physiotherapists in the 'prescription' of exercise for particular ailments and, resonating with neoliberal imperatives, are sometimes seen as a cheaper alternative. Exercise is framed in terms of diagnosis and treatment, explicitly so in the EiM movement, and trainers manifestly compare themselves with health workers, even describing themselves as 'doctors in this field' (Hutson 2013: 67). Writ large therefore are the contradictory processes of the medicalization of sport and exercise and the weakening of medical power through areas of convergence between the fitness industry and medicine.

Sport, medicine and health: a conceptual framework

As much as the literature reviewed illustrates a connection between medicine, health and sport/fitness, two core gaps in our conceptual understanding remain. First the interdependence of the paradigmatic, institutional and interactional levels is under-explored. The micro-sociological embodied experiences of exercise and sports participation have certainly seen the quest for exciting significance alter in line with changing notions of health, which stem from broader macro-structural changes to the delivery and discourse of medicine. However, in the final analysis (of fitness), medicine is afforded a relatively peripheral position, or at least only operative at the level of public health narrative. These accounts largely subsume PAHP within the broader discourse of NPH, without examining the similarities and differences, convergence and incongruence. A consequence of this is the false homogenization of medicine through the obfuscation of intra-medical conflicts and interests and, ultimately, the depiction of medicalization processes as monolithic, inexorable and irreversible. In the process, both sports medical actors, and indeed para-medical specialities such as sports physiotherapy, are written out of the account. Any analysis of the interdependence of sport, medicine and health which neither recognizes a distinct medical specialism of sports medicine nor the system of professions in which it is located, must necessarily be partial. An understanding of the interdependence of these different dimensions is essential.

Second, the works discussed above focus rather more on fitness than sport. Accepting them uncritically can therefore replicate the conflation of sport and exercise identified as a fundamentally problematic aspect of the sport–health ideology (see Chapter 1). Crossley (2006) notes that some gym goers take part in sport, and some even join the gym to rehabilitate from sports injury, but the spatial location of his ethnography restricts a more holistic exploration of their social experience. Lupton (1995: 148) makes a more explicit attempt to distinguish between play- and body maintenance-oriented physical activities, but in failing to fully interrogate this distinction ultimately projects health and the emotional experience inherent in sport (conceived of as the quest for excitement, see below) as a 'complex admixture' of motives for participation, rather than inherently conflicting phenomena. Moreover, the centrality of the commercial sport sector in these narratives only partially reflects the breadth of sports provision in Western nations. In disproportionately focusing on *intended* consequences of a discrete range of activities, the analysis reproduces rather than expands upon the impact of the ideology of healthism.

The implications of a more rounded, nuanced consideration of sport-related activities can be seen in the work of Scambler *et al.* (2004). They argue that the health–sport relationship has become increasingly paradoxical as identity construction has become both more important and more complex in contemporary societies. Specifically, 'the price paid for looking and feeling good, and therefore looking and feeling healthy ... may be health risk or even declining health status' (Scambler *et al.* 2004: 112). The necessity to construct identities and the constraints in which identities are constructed mean that, 'people are increasingly seduced by the hypercommodification of either sport [perhaps more accurately exercise] which is conducive to health longevity or sport which is injurious to health and longevity' (Scambler *et al.* 2004: 119). Elite athletes chosen as national representatives on the basis of their physical excellence, pushing the limits of human performance and establishing new world records, are symbols of national health, and thus indicative of the possibilities of individual health. They are, and they perpetuate, the physical embodiment of the sport–health ideology.

Sport, medicine, health and Elias

The conceptual framework underpinning this text is perhaps best described as an Eliasian-informed synthesis of the above ideas. While this perspective has significantly but thus far mostly implicitly shaped the discussion, a few further conceptual clarifications are required.

Commitment to exploring the interdependence of the various manifestations of sport and 'sport-like' activities resonates with Elias' figurational or process sociological approach. Elias, along with Bourdieu, was 'virtually alone among major sociologists … to have written seriously on sports' (Bourdieu and Wacquant 1992: 93) and, as prior reference to the quest for excitement (Elias and Dunning 1986) illustrates, he did so by considering sport in relation to leisure forms more broadly. For Elias, sport-related research was 'as significant to our understanding of the development of European societies as it is for that of sport itself' (Elias 1986a: 127). Contemporary trends have meant that the separation of studies of medicine and health and sport is no longer sustainable.

Second, Elias's concept of the figuration 'invokes "the individual", "agency", "society", "social change", "power" and "structure" simultaneously but purposely without being reducible to any of these components' (Dunning and Hughes 2013: 52). Consequently, it enables us to more adequately conceptualize the relationships between discourse, practice and identity in medicalization processes. Via 'figuration', Elias sought to emphasize interdependence; 'since people are more or less dependent upon each other first by nature and then through social learning … and socially generated reciprocal needs they exist … only in pluralities' (Elias 2000: 482). Consequently all social relations are both enabling and constraining and any notion of power requires identifying relations in a historically situated context and between multiple parties. For instance, in his study of established–outsider relations (Elias and Scotson 1994), Elias exemplified how networks of interdependence, consolidated by a groups' length of association and use of 'praise' and 'blame gossip' to construct a 'group charisma' (of the established) or 'group disgrace' (of the outsiders), augmented traditional aspects of social power such as economic resources and occupational prestige. Such contextual specificities to sports medicine's development are crucial to understanding the dynamics of practice, interprofessional relations in sports healthcare and contemporary manifestations of PAHP. The analysis of sports medicine practice needs to figurationally locate clinicians, positioning doctors both as wielders of power in interpersonal relationships and as actors influenced by the broader network of relationships in which they are enmeshed, thus illustrating how such agency and structural components are fundamentally intertwined (Elias, 1978). Intended and unintended consequences comingle due to the inability of any group or individual to act autonomously. De Swaan's notion of reluctant imperialism is underpinned by this conceptualization, and the deployment of the concept of medicalization in this book derives from a sensitivity towards the polymorphous and polyvalent character of power. Here we explore the ebb and flow of social processes as human interdependence operates in multiple, complex and frequently unanticipated ways.

Third, Elias's concept of civilizing processes helps us to frame social developments in the perceptions of the role and value of the body. Simply stated, Elias argued that, over time, people were increasingly expected to exert greater self-regulation over their bodies, with manners, emotional expression and bodily deportment increasingly important to the stratification of social groups. Thus, the aesthetically healthy body has become 'a designer commodity, which can be purchased by those with sufficient resources ... [yet] also a moral achievement, because you have to purchase it with your own labour' (Porter 1999, p. 312). The 'differential acquisition of new forms of self-control' not only enables social stratification based on corporeal appearance, but facilitates the blame or praise of individuals relative to their (in-)ability to conform (Stuiz, 2011). Pace Lupton (1995), Elias's notion of civilized bodies provides greater explanatory purchase for the focus and direction of Foucauldian notions of disciplinary power and surveillance. Moreover, what has been termed Elias's 'central theory', *The Civilizing Process*, provides 'analysis of the historical development of emotions and psychological life ... in relation to the connections ... with larger scale processes such as state formation, urbanisation and economic development' (van Krieken 1998: 353). In so doing it extrapolates from the principles of figurations to: (a) give priority to the analysis of developmental processes; and (b) bridge the macro-micro sociological divide, or research which focuses upon a particularly high generality of understanding (e.g. the construction of health policy) and research which focuses on the minutiae of everyday life (e.g. illness experience).

Fourth, Elias's sociology of knowledge provides an important tool for understanding the development of 'ideologies' and, particularly in this context, those such as *the health imperative*, NPH and PAHP. Following the logic of *The Civilizing Process*, Elias (1987) argued that over time human knowledge has become less influenced by immediate self-interest, egocentrism and strong emotions and, correlatively, humans have increasingly enhanced their capacity to distance themselves from their objects of study and become reflexive about their role as producers of knowledge. Elias considered the structural factors that enabled the natural sciences (e.g. medicine) to ascend the epistemological hierarchy and linked this to the historical and contextual specificities in which particular types of human knowledge are generated. Eschewing philosophical debates about truth and social construction, he explored the balance/blend of involvement (self-interest, emotion, etc.) and detachment (distanciation, reflexivity, etc.) to illustrate how ideas exist/persist not according to an external, preordained logic, but in conjunction with the emotional gratification they evoke, and thus only if they survive 'reality testing ... in the crucible of experience' (Elias 1987: 56). Correlatively Goudsblom (1986) notes that the development of public health is not simply about the development of science, but is reminiscent of what Elias (2000: 365–379) described as the 'social constraint towards self-constraint' and the concomitant development of 'delicacy of feeling'. For Goudsblom the heightened valorization of physical health in the twentieth century was due to processes of individualization and democratization, with 'the individual ... [increasingly] compelled to regulate his [sic] conduct in an increasingly differentiated, more even and more stable manner' (Elias 2000: 367). As technological developments lead expectations of longevity to be experienced by larger proportions of the population, so these behavioural norms become more widely diffused.

Thus, health, like civilizing processes, is intimately entwined with the way human beings live in and through their bodies, assumptions of what people should and should not look like, the expectations that people have of themselves and others in their interpersonal relations and the allocation of social status through praise and/or shame. The manifestation of human control over the social body shifts over time and in relation to the broader structural context of human production, such that in times of nutritional scarcity physical size is synonymous with social status, while in times of abundance status is more closely associated with slenderness. Fundamentally then, 'health is a corporeal problem of control', which is underpinned by 'questions about the relationship between external regulation of individual and collective bodies and internalized self-control of behaviour and emotion' (Malcolm and Mansfield 2013: 409). The rise of surveillance medicine, which has helped deconstruct the health-illness binary and thus placed each individual's health-status on a continuum, both centres and validates Elias' emphasis on an explicitly relational sociology. The identification of disease pre-cursors and the introduction of interventions based on risk assessment means that human health becomes inherently a question of one of Elias's central tenets, interdependence; of the individual's life expectancy relative to population norms. The development of modern medicine is a project predicated on the desire to render the human body and its various functions more malleable, more rationalized. The development of healthcare within the broader welfare state stems from the growing awareness of our fundamental interdependence as a population and the impact of oneself upon others (de Swaan 1988). State provision of healthcare essentially represents an extension of the external regulation of intimate embodied lives to render them more predictable and controllable. We therefore begin our analysis of sport-medicine-health relations with the development of sports medicine as a discrete yet state-mandated and licensed medical specialism.

Chapter 3

The development of sports medicine

Early iterations of sports medicine are as old as medicine itself. The Ancient Greek physician Herodicus has been described as the father of sports medicine (Georgoulis *et al.* 2007). His most notable pupil, Hippocrates (460–370 BC), argued that exercise contributed to the balancing of the four humours: blood; phlegm; black bile; and yellow bile. Galen (AD 130–200) included rest/motion (exercise) amongst the 'six things non-natural' which, in moderation, would optimize good health (the others being air, diet, sleep/awake, excretions/retentions and passions of the mind). Conversely both he and Hippocrates were critical of the immoderate lifestyle of elite athletes (Dunn *et al.* 2007). Although the humoral theory of medicine was superseded by new medical paradigms in the intervening millennia, the restriction of sports medicine to prophylactic measures essentially remained static until the late nineteenth century because, quite simply, there were few known effective cures. Exercise was advocated for the treatment of a number of specific ailments – e.g. gout, consumption – but the prescription for injuries incurred during sport was simply to rest (Berryman 2010).

The range of sport, medicine and health intersections identified during the nineteenth century defies the evidence for the efficacy of exercise. Prominent themes include the role of sport and exercise in: the development of manliness and morality; countering physical deterioration as a consequence of urbanization; improving the health of factory workers and, at times of conflict and war, the wider population; and in relation to eugenics and social Darwinism (including race issues) (Welshman 1998). In addition, there are detailed accounts of the relationship between medicine and the restriction of sport and exercise opportunities for females due to fears of the negative impact on health in general, and childbearing in particular (e.g. Lenskyj 1986; Park 2015; Vertinsky 1990). Ultimately however, these accounts serve to reinforce our understanding of the sport–health ideology rather than explore sports medicine more broadly. As Cronin (2007: 24) points out, this literature 'has concentrated not so much on sports medicine as a practice that treats injury, but more on the broad development of ideas that linked health and well-being to the pursuit of physical activity'.

As noted in Chapter 1, the accepted sociological interpretation of the development of sports medicine is that it has been driven by performance concerns; that by the end of the twentieth century, physiology had 'been put in the service of sport' (Hoberman 1992: 74). Yet in examining the specialism in relation to the professional traits discussed in Chapter 2, we see that the medicalization of sport has been far less smooth or unilinear than this narrative depicts. There has been international variation in terms of intra- and inter-professional conflicts and in the deployment of essentially contradictory jurisdictional claims. At times, doctors have striven for greater social influence through medical and state recognition, and at times they have been cajoled into action by sporting authorities.

Consequently, the focus of this chapter is the institutional manifestation of sports medicine; that is, its emergence as a 'profession', and the relationship between this professional group and medicalization processes. It provides a cross-cultural comparison of attempts to embark on 'professional projects', explores the internal and external conflicts which in various contexts were counter to the development of the specialism, and identifies the reluctant imperialism (de Swaan 1989) evident in relation to certain issues. It concludes by focusing on the 'professionalization' of British sports medicine, a case which both exemplifies the changing social conceptions of health discussed in Chapter 2 and is most central to the subsequent analysis. The value of this focus can be clarified through a brief review of what has now become the orthodox historical account of the development of sports medicine.

Professional traits and sports medicine

As we previously saw, a profession might be defined as a distinct occupational group, authoritative in its fields, organizationally coherent, and able to control its own membership and direct the activities of those in related fields. To what extent have these traits been evident in the development of sports medicine?

Sports medicine established a degree of organizational coherence in 1928 when a meeting was convened at the St. Moritz Winter Olympics. Attended by 50 physicians associated with 11 nations competing at the games (Pfister 2011), the meeting resolved to found the Association Internationale Medico Sportive, which in turn changed its name to Fédération Internationale de Médecine Sportive (FIMS) in 1934. FIMS has been organized into linguistic and regional subgroupings (currently consisting of eight multinational and four continental organizations), and its membership has grown considerably in recent years, from a reported 55 member states in 1979 (Williams 1979), to 83 in 1989 and 141 in March 2016.

Box 3.1 Foundation dates for selected national sports medicine associations

German Society for Sports Medicine and Prevention	1912
Netherlands Association of Sports Medicine	1922
Swiss Society for Sports Medicine	1923
Italian Sports Medicine Association	1929
Polish Sports Medicine Association	1937
Sociedad Uruguaya de Medicina del Deporte	1941
Japanese Federation of Physical Fitness and Sports Medicine	1949
Swedish Association of Sports Medicine	1952
British Association of Sport and Medicine	1952
American College of Sports Medicine	1954
Sports Medicine Australia	1963
Canadian Academy of Sport Medicine	1970

Source: www.ismj.com/pages/311417173/FIMS/Associations/fimsmemberassociations. asp accessed 10 February 2015, supplemented with data from Carter (2012a).

Prior to this, Germany had been one of a small number of countries in which a national sports medicine organization had been established. While Carter (2012b) and FIMS cite 1912 as a foundation date for German sports medicine, Hoberman (1992) and Pfister (2011) focus on 1924 and the foundation of the Deutscher Ärztebund zur Förderung der Leibesügungen (the German Medical Association for the Advancement of Physical Activities or DÄB). Undoubtedly, however, Germany did lead the world in establishing laboratories for the evaluation of athletes and mechanisms for the dissemination of sports medicine knowledge. This is not to say that individuals self-identifying as sports doctors had not appeared in other countries at this time. For instance Matlock House in Manchester became known as the 'Footballers' Hospital' in the late nineteenth century due to its sports-centric treatments and clientele (Carter 2007). Similarly sport-related work was being conducted at the Carnegie Nutrition Laboratory in the 1910s (Berryman 2012) and Adolphe Abrahams attended the 1912 Olympic Games as the official medical officer for British athletics (Carter 2012b). However, outside of Germany sports medicine essentially comprised 'an abundance of disaggregated practice' (Heggie 2011: 26). A Swiss physician was elected the first president of FIMS, but infrastructural advantages made Germany the obvious choice to locate the secretariat.

The organizational coherence of sports medicine was initially restricted by conceptual, disciplinary and spatial differences. First, sports medicine 'suffered' due to its variable and amorphous definition. While medical sub-disciplines tend to focus on particular technical interventions (e.g. surgery, anaesthesiology), organs/organ systems (cardiology, nephrology), physical states (oncology, obstetrics), or the health issues of particular demographic groups (paediatrics, occupational and environmental medicine), sports medicine 'is an extremely unpromising field to convert into a medical specialism' (Heggie 2010a: 458). Elite sports medicine essentially serves a particular demographic group (see Chapter 7), but the ubiquity of sport and exercise makes participants' experiences, ranging from quasi professional performance to exercise in the pursuit of health and, increasingly, exercise for rehabilitative purposes, remarkably diverse. Moreover, other branches of medicine (see below) lay claim to the treatment of sport-induced conditions and so undermine any notion of sports medicine as definitive. In contrast to medicine per se, the goals and parameters of which were more precise, concise and widely accepted, sports medicine was conceptually slippery, contested and ultimately lacking in distinction.

Second, the leading sports medicine specialists of the early twentieth century were drawn from various medical disciplines (Pfister 2011; Heggie 2011). For instance, football trainers who occupied an influential position in sports medicine from *circa* 1885, drew on technical roots derived from 'unorthodox alternative medicine' (Carter 2009a: 261). This led to fundamental tensions between medical and 'lay' treatment, with debates centring on the relative merits of experimental (medical) and experiential (lay) knowledge, and the respective roles of physiological and performance outcomes in the evaluation of treatment efficacy. The blurring of sports medicine and sports science – to some extent the kind of pure versus applied distinction we explore in Chapter 7 – compounded this. Consequently, sports medicine consisted of 'an intricate network of enthusiasts and semi-specialists some medically trained, some amateurs, who participated in and created a network of health beliefs; some of these had long, traditional roots, while others were interpretations of cutting edge medical research' (Heggie 2011: 50).

Third, in that sports medicine was practised in a variety of contexts, (laboratories, private clinics, tracks, pitches and occasionally hospitals) it pre-empted the spatiality of surveillance medicine in reaching into the community (Armstrong 1995). However, because it did so without having first established significant social influence, spatial dispersion and an essentially unregulated commercial environment retarded sports medicine's coherence. While medical practitioners more closely aligned to university-based science sought to establish expertise through knowledge dissemination, those who literally and/or metaphorically experimented in the field – trainers with professional sports teams, Harley Street specialists – undermined their market position if they sought to share knowledge (cf. Johnson 1972).

Thus, development of an authoritative and definitive voice faltered because sports medicine's focus was poorly delineated and its members were ideologically, physically and economically divided. The impact of these factors has been enduring. Williams and Sperryn (1976: ix) define sports medicine as, 'an integrated multi-disciplinary field embracing the relevant areas of clinical medicine (sports traumatology, the medicine of sport and sports psychiatry) and the appropriate allied scientific disciplines (including physiology, psychology and biomechanics)'. Ryan's (1989: 13) conception is of an even broader field, such that sports medicine practitioners may include, 'physicians, coaches, trainers, exercise physiologists, psychologists, sociologists, physical educators and others whose special interests are less well-defined'.

A further feature of the definitional distinctiveness of this field is the value placed on practical sporting experience. First evident in the policies of DÄB in the 1920s (Pfister 2011), it continues today. For instance, Ken Kennedy, a doctor and former player, concludes a list of the 'ideal' qualities of the rugby club doctor (e.g. knowledge of traumatology and the kinesiology of rugby; experience of rehabilitation and orthopaedics; good referral contacts; the ability to effectively liaise with physiotherapists) with the claim that, '*most importantly* the doctor should have an affinity for the game and the people in it' (Kennedy 1990: 315, emphasis added). While such statements are attempts to claim 'a mark of distinction from other doctors' (Pfister 2011: 283), they stem from an *in*ability to monopolize more conventional markers of professional status, such as technical expertise or esoteric skill. Indeed, this kind of democratization of knowledge is frequently identified as a challenge to medical dominance (see Chapter 2). Notably, 'a requirement of personal experience as a patient [is] not applied to any other medical specialism' (Heggie 2010a: 459).

Box 3.2 Mission Statement, Fédération Internationale de Médecine du Sport

- To promote the study and development of sports medicine throughout the world.
- To preserve and improve the health of mankind through physical fitness and sports participation.
- To scientifically study the natural and pathological implications of physical training and sports participation.
- To organise and/or sponsor internationally based scientific meetings, courses, congresses, and exhibits in the field of sports medicine.
- To cooperate with national and international organisations in sports medicine and related fields.
- To publish scientific information in the field of sports medicine and other related fields.

Source: www.fims.org/about/ Accessed 10 February 2015.

But a deeper and more fundamental tension exists within sports medicine; the contrasting and potentially contradictory goals of health and performance. As we saw in Chapter 2, while medicine has evolved to be much more than simply the relief of suffering, the explicit nature of this tension makes sports medicine different by degree, if not in absolute terms. For example, according to the FIMS website, the organization 'aims primarily to promote the study and development of sports medicine throughout the world, and to *assist athletes in achieving optimal performance* by maximising their genetic potential, health, nutrition, and high-quality medical care and training' (FIMS 2015, emphasis added). However, this prioritization of 'performance' is directly at odds with the emphasis on *health* contained in FIMS' mission statement (see Box 3.2). While the health–performance tension is an ever-present consideration, the exact outcome of deliberations varies. Some national organizations (e.g. Japan) explicitly embraced health from the outset while others (e.g. Australia) still do not formally incorporate it in their title. If the move towards 'professional' status is not solely predicated on developing certain traits, but dependent on the ability of a group to persuade other powerful groups to recognize and validate what they do, the development of sports medicine cannot simply be a seamless and unilinear development oriented towards performance in the rationalistic pursuit of human excellence. To illustrate this we need to explore the nationally specific professional projects that have been pursued in sports medicine.

Professional projects in sports medicine

The medicalization of sport in terms of the institutionalization of sports medicine belies considerable international diversity. Here we compare four such examples: pre-War Germany; post-1945 East Germany (GDR) and the USSR; the USA; and Canada. These show that globally there have been different degrees to which national associations have embarked upon an explicit and intentional 'professional project' (Larson 1977), and different emphases on health and performance in each.

Pre-war Germany

As noted, the earliest, most explicit and perhaps most successful attempt to construct a sports medicine profession was in Germany (Hoberman 1992; Pfister 2011). There were early tensions with Arthur Mallwitz leading the call for a performance-oriented sports medicine, and Georg Nicolai seeking to locate the specialism within a broader public health discourse. However, following the aforementioned establishment of DÄB (1924) disputes seemed to dissipate behind more unified objectives for the profession. Limiting membership to registered physicians (plus a few nominated honorary members) enhanced disciplinary coherence. Despite such exclusionary measures, DÄB membership reached 3000 by 1933.

The DÄB professional project included facilitating information exchange through meetings and conferences (Pfister 2011). While an independent journal was not economically viable, DÄB successfully sequestered dedicated sections of more established medical journals to disseminate sports medicine knowledge. It sought to develop international cooperation evident in its role in the establishment of FIMS. It strove to identify a distinct jurisdictional domain consisting of research (encompassing health education, sport injuries and performance sport), professional practice and policy. The latter included the failure to establish 'sports physician' as a regulated title but the successful definition of a 'quasi-specialist' role with specified training, occupational experience and sports participation as prerequisites for GPs who wished to identify as sports physicians. DÄB claimed schools, higher education, public health and exercise facilities (gyms, tracks, etc.) as sports medicine's rightful domains. In terms of practice, DÄB set up advice centres designed to provide medical supervision to all sports participants. While finance restricted their growth, there were 15 such centres in Berlin by 1930. Thus, although DÄB focused on the traditional foundations of professional status, crucially it 'chose a path which was to ensure its control of sports medicine without arousing the opposition of [existing] doctors' associations' (Pfister 2011: 287).

GDR and USSR

The communist sports medicine systems of Cold War Europe (1945–1990) built on these foundations. The proportion of Olympic medals won by athletes from Eastern European communist countries increased from 29% in 1952 to 57% in 1976 and, given the economies and populations relative to Western states, this success was widely attributed to sports medicine. The dominant nations were the GDR and USSR. While the broader structure of power between the nations meant that the two systems aligned as the 'Soviet sports medicine system was more or less transplanted to the GDR' (Riordan 1987: 21), the traditions of technical skill and organizational coherence gave the GDR system considerable leverage. Sports medicine only received Russian state recognition in 1977.

Under this system each region and district had its own sports medicine centre, which provided sport-related health screening to the general population and licensed participation in sport. This provision dovetailed with support for elite athletes, which included talent screening; regular health surveillance including tests to evaluate training effects; coach and athlete education; sport-specific medical teams to support competition and training; specialist hospitals for more significant interventions; and dedicated provision for female and child athletes. While there was some reluctance amongst the broader medical community to accept sports medicine as a specialism, and contestation over resourcing, the alignment of sports medicine with nationalist goals, and the nature of centrally-planned societies, meant that discordance was either short lived or muted (Riordan 1987).

USA

The American case illustrates the obverse of the professionalization spectrum. Here, the coalition of medicine and physical education provided a 'distinct and unique heritage' (Berryman 2012: 43). These relationships were evident from the 1880s, with 11 of the first 12 Presidents of the American Association for the Advancement of Physical Education having trained as medical doctors (Berryman 2010), and in 1954 the foundation of the ACSM (American College of Sports Medicine). An explicitly multidisciplinary body organized around three core constituencies (medicine, basic and applied science, allied health and education), founding members were drawn from physical education (eight individuals, four of whom were physiologists) and medicine (three cardiologists). There were clear signs of deference to the social status of medicine. Even though the American Heart Association (AHA) and American College of Cardiology (ACC) rejected/ignored requests to play a more central role in the establishment of the ACSM, their members played a disproportionally prominent role in the administration of the organization. Ultimately, the professed belief that these multiple skill sets needed combining because no one profession (physiologists, cardiologists or physical educationalists) possessed definitive knowledge, led to the ACSM's formation. Because it contained few orthopaedists or team doctors, the treatment of sports injuries was never a major preoccupation and the development of performance medicine largely took place outside the ACSM. Rather, 'it was their interest and research in exercise, cardiovascular disease and youth fitness' that stimulated the ACSM's formation (Berryman 2012: 43). These goals seem to have minimized inter-professional conflict within sports medicine in the US.

Conversely the definitive and authoritative status of the ACSM has continually faced intra-medical professional challenge. In the same year that the ACSM was formed, the AMA established a committee on injuries in sport which, in 1959, became a standing committee for the Medical Aspects of Sport. In 1962, the American Academy of Orthopaedic Surgeons founded a Committee on Sports Medicine and in 1975 the American Orthopaedic Society for Sports Medicine was established. The American Academy of Pediatrics and the American Academy of Family Physicians also have committees on sports medicine. In 1991, *Physician and Sports Medicine* reported that there were 82 different groups in the US who considered themselves involved in the delivery of some form of sports medicine (cited in Waddington 1996). The founding of the seemingly tautological American Medical Society for Sports Medicine in this year reveals the conflicts over jurisdictional dominance. Indeed, the ACSM has explicitly eschewed a professional project until recently perhaps (and the launch of EiM, see Chapter 4). Indeed, in 1968 the ACSM pronounced that sports medicine is 'a perspective' and that 'there is no single profession to be defined for sports medicine' (cited in Safai 2007: 323). Inter-professional collaboration within the ACSM has been achieved against a background of intra-medical conflict over the sports medicine domain.

Canada

Our final example, Canadian sports medicine, was centrally driven by per-formance concerns but largely in response to East European sports medi-cine. In the 1950s, attempts to establish a Canadian branch of FIMS were positioned within a public health discourse. Leading advocate, Doris Plewes, made no explicit appeal to the professional sport community and sought, instead, to challenge what she saw as the widespread *mis*concep-tion of sports medicine as primarily concerned with elite performance. But, at this time, the health rationale was insufficient, perhaps because the notion of health was less all-embracing than it is today or perhaps because the sport–health ideology was so fundamentally unchallenged. Rather, it was the twin Olympic experiences of Mexico 1968 and Montreal 1976 that facilitated the institutionalization of Canadian sports medicine (Safai 2007). In part, the Mexico games were marked by concerns over the effects on the competitive success of Canadian athletes of holding the games at altitude (see next section), but more significantly a post-games 'taskforce' served to highlight the relatively limited medical support for Canadian athletes; two doctors (one competing in the games) and two physiothera-pists (one full, one part-time), compared with the nine doctors and 18 trainers available to one, unnamed, national rival (Safai 2007).

This experience galvanized Canadian authorities to enhance, standard-ize and thus 'professionalize' the provision of sports medicine. The Cana-dian Olympic Association Medical Advisory Committee, the Canadian Athletic Therapists Association and the Canadian Association of Sports Sciences (CASS) had been established in 1959, 1965 and 1966 respec-tively, but post-Mexico saw the formalization of the Canadian Academy of Sport Medicine (CASM) (1970) and a separate body for sports physio-therapy (1972). The subsequent establishment of 'Game Plan 76' in the run up to the Montreal Olympics led to Canada's first integrated sports medicine team. *Sport Canada* formed The Sport Medicine and Science Council of Canada (SMSCC) to enable the coordination of interested groups. Government provided funding because 'doing so was compatible with the agenda of producing excellence ... [in] high performance sport' (Safai 2007: 326).

The institutionalization of sport medicine created three areas of inter-professional competition: representation on the SMSCC, selection for medical teams deployed at major games, and legitimate scope of practice for the respective healthcare therapies (Safai 2005). Safai's (2005: 99) account illustrates how, in deploying administrative resources to increase membership, for instance, occupational groups used the committee 'as a platform on which to boost and accelerate their professional project'. Furthermore, Safai detects jurisdictional tensions between competing healthcare providers within this system of professions, with debates centred on knowledge, expertise and professional accreditation. Despite medicine's dominance, CASM's definitive and authoritative status was undermined by the demands of clients or user groups that shaped the relative influence of different providers (see Chapters 7 and 8). The outcome of these divisions, plus funding issues and competition with provincial councils, led to the dissolution of the SMSCC in the late 1990s.

Understanding professional projects in sports medicine

The central conclusion from this comparative analysis is that there is no single trope that can summarize the medicalization of sport in this institutional sense. We can see distinct national patterns of 'professionalization' within sports medicine. There is no doubt that the link between performance and national prestige, as Hoberman (1992) and Waddington (1996) argue, has been and remains a significant impetus. For instance, ever since 1932, when Olympic host cities started to centrally provide medical services there have been attempts not 'to be outdone' by previous hosts (Heggie 2011: 76). Similarly, Riordan (1987: 20) notes that the desire for better medical support in the build-up to the LA Olympics (1984) led the USOC to form committees for Sports Medicine and for Sports Equipment and Technology, while Canadian commitment to high performance sports medicine was renewed in the run up to hosting the Vancouver Winter Olympics in 2010, through the *Own the Podium* programme (Safai 2007). But as the early German and Canadian cases show, these developments can be largely autonomous of the commercialization and politicization of sport. The American example further shows that sports medicine can become nationally established with almost no reference to sport performance.

The role of 'sport' in the development of sports medicine

Sports medicine physicians have pursued various negotiations with other branches of medicine and the state to establish professional, specialist status. Yet as the literature on professions and medicalization shows (see

Chapter 2), relations with clients are also centrally important in shaping medicine's relative power and influence. In this section, we look at sports medicine's relations with two other institutional 'clients': the IOC and boxing authorities. The former shows the potential conflict between sport and medicalization/professionalization processes. The latter highlights the divisions within medicine, which explain how medical imperialism is at times 'reluctant' (de Swaan 1989).

The IOC Medical Commission

Widely respected for being at the vanguard of contemporary sports medicine issues, initially the IOC exhibited a considerable desire for independence from medicine. For instance, from 1960 to 1964, it would only consult sports medicine when it 'found it absolutely necessary' (Wrynn 2004: 214). In this, the IOC were enabled by a small number of medically-trained executive committee members. For instance, Dr Arthur Porritt led the IOC's first subcommittee on doping, and 'recommended that the IOC not involve itself too deeply in questions of science and medicine' (Wrynn 2004: 213). However, the combination of altitude, drugs and gender testing, which converged at the Mexico Olympics, exposed the limitations of the IOC's medical expertise and fundamentally altered relations between sport and medicine forever.

The prospect of competing at altitude involved questions about specialist training which, in turn, related to amateurism regulations. Thus, these issues were as political as they were scientific (Heggie 2008). While Wrynn (2004: 217), for example, argued that the IOC 'dealt with the problem of altitude by virtually ignoring much of the scientific evidence', Heggie (2008: 228) detected 'a compromise between the physiological demands of altitude and the administrative and financial demands of amateurism'. Either way, it is clear that sport could operate a relatively high degree of independence when issues relating to athletes' health created opportunities for greater medicalization.

The greater dependence of the IOC in relation to doping and sex testing (see also Chapter 10) entailed a different set of tensions. Indeed, in 1961, IOC President Avery Brundage had insisted that the organization needed medical advice and 'more competent' structures to determine how to define doping (cited in Wrynn 2004: 218). This issue precipitated the establishment of the IOC Medical Commission in 1967, only two of whose founders were IOC members. One of them, Porritt, now endorsed the incorporation of external expertise. The IOC Medical Commission immediately assumed responsibility for drug testing and at its second meeting announced the sex testing procedures for the Mexico games. These developments divided (sports) medicine. The president of FIMS argued for the greater role of medicine and others questioned the efficacy of the proposed testing programme (Wrynn 2004). IOC leaders were uncomfortable with the influence ceded to medical 'outsiders'. After Mexico, Brundage tried to rein in the Medical Commission, arguing that they met too frequently. In 1972, his successor, Lord Killanin, suggested that the Commission was too large.

The example of the IOC Medical Commission shows that it was not just the search for performance-enhancement that drove the development of sports medicine, but also the demands of policing participation. Here, sports organizations were able to show a greater degree of autonomy. However, what sports organizations could *not* control was the broader cultural discourse that positioned medicine as the arbiter of social issues (deviancy) and an effective tool of social control. Conversely, where developments were driven by the needs of powerful sporting institutions (i.e. drug and gender testing) there was considerable potential for them to divide the medical community. This latter point is particularly well illustrated in relation to boxing.

Boxing and medicine

Debates about the health dangers of boxing started in *The Lancet* in 1893 (Sheard 1998). Initially, objections centred on moral rather than medical grounds, with some early deaths in boxing attributed to emotional states (over-excitement and anxiety) rather than the damage inflicted to the brain by punches. One reason for this stance was medical uncertainty over causation, particularly as symptoms often occurred long after boxing contests finished. Even though the term 'punch drunk' (introduced in 1928) drew attention to the link between the sport and brain damage, debates in the journal showed a divided community and an agnostic editorship.

Albeit in response to ethical and medical objections, the medicalization of boxing was largely driven by the sport's administrators. The National Sporting Club had long required boxers to undergo a medical examination (Carter 2009a), but to placate boxing's growing number of critics the British Board of Boxing Control (BBBC) appointed a Chief Medical Officer (1946) and established a national medical committee (1950). The increased medical surveillance of boxers during the early 1950s saw them routinely examined before and after each bout, and a doctor within call *during* each bout. Medicine became centrally implicated both in the instruction of tournament officials and trainers, and the licensing and insurance of boxers (Welshman 1998).

Boxing faced increasing, and increasingly forceful, critique. While initial challenges came from 'solitary researchers' (Welshman 1998: 10) they subsequently became more coordinated: a leader article in the *British Medical Journal* in 1954; the parliamentary activism of Dr Edith Summerskill; and the Royal College of Physicians (RCP) commissioned the 'Roberts Report'

(1969). But the lack of conclusive scientific evidence available (until the 1970s) meant that these debates were 'a broader ideological struggle about courage, masculinity, the British character, sadism and the dangerous nature of all sport' (Sheard 1998: 86). Debates embraced the qualitative distinction between amateur and professional boxing, and the civilizing influence on young people potentially diverted from deviant lifestyles. The efforts of people such as Blondstein and Clarke, honorary medical officers to the Amateur Boxing Association (ABA), were important to the sport's defence. Sports medicine's pro-boxing lobby argued that evidence largely related to the historic lack of regulation and, subsequently, that (increased) medical supervision was required to minimize the dangers of boxing. Paradoxically the challenge (some) medical personnel posed to the very existence of boxing created the conditions that led boxing to become increasingly medicalized.

The largely moral nature of arguments over the legitimacy of boxing, and the role of medicine within these debates, could be interpreted as medical imperialism. But these events also highlight the 'internal divisions and intra-professional jealousies' (Sheard 1998: 98), which meant that medicine could never present a united front. Indeed, Welshman interpreted these developments as, 'an interesting illustration of the weaknesses of the medical establishment, exposing the divisions that exist between medical specialisms, individual doctors and rival bodies' (Welshman 1998: 13). As medical knowledge advanced, 'doctors were increasingly *drawn into* [boxing-related] court cases' (Welshman 1998: 6, emphasis added) and so were called upon to adjudicate on social conflicts. Clearly an example of medicalization, *pace* de Swaan (1989), it was essentially reluctant imperialism and, in this respect, it contrasts with the more recent, explicit attempt to medicalize concussion injuries, as explored in Chapter 9.

The development of sports medicine in Britain

Contrary to the thesis that places the rational pursuit of performance as the driving force in a somewhat unilinear development, we have seen that professionalization has been retarded by sports medicine's conceptual, disciplinary and spatial divisions. There is, moreover, considerable variation in the degree to which sports medicine physicians have pursued professional projects and/or been 'successful' in those pursuits. Sports medicine has not only sought to negotiate a role in relation to the state and other branches of medicine, but has had uneasy and contradictory relations with the varying demands/needs of sports organizations. In the final section of this chapter, we explore the development of sports medicine in Britain. This is vital for the contextualization of much of the subsequent analysis in this book, but it is also highly illustrative in its own right. The different goals, networks of interdependency, power relations, and performance–health dynamics in this example provide additional explanatory purchase for the medicalization of sport.

The inaugural meeting that led to the foundation of the British Association of Sport and Medicine (BASM) took place in 1952. Founder member Adolphe Abrahams expressed the desire for BASM 'to advise on all the general principles of athletic training and sports-related medical injuries and to conduct research into sports injuries' (cited in Carter 2012b: 58). Consequently BASM's claim to specialist status was far more oriented to performance than public health matters. BASM affiliated to FIMS in 1954, published a *Bulletin* in 1967, which in turn became the *British Journal of Sports Medicine* (BJSM) in 1968, and from the early 1980s saw the introduction of various, but ad-hoc, attempts to establish recognized specialist qualifications. These educational initiatives were boosted in 1994 when the Royal Society of Medicine established a sports medicine section, and again in 1998 when the Intercollegiate Academic Board of Sport and Exercise Medicine (IABSEM) was formed to enhance the standardization of provision (itself superseded by the Faculty of Sport and Exercise Medicine (FSEM) in 2006). The IABSEM began work on an application for specialist status in 2003, and 'Sport and Exercise Medicine' became a formally recognized medical speciality in the UK in 2005 (Heggie 2010a: 473). The Institute of Sport and Exercise Medicine became the research arm of the FSEM in 2007 (Jones *et al.* 2011). Accordingly, BASM changed its name in 1999 to incorporate 'exercise'; hence BASEM.

In assembling these professional 'traits', British sports medicine was constrained by a number of factors. Dogged by the definitional issues that affect the specialism more generally, the professional project of British sports medicine was also restricted by personnel matters. Although BASM began as a primarily physician-based body, low membership numbers necessitated sacrificing coherence and social status for critical mass. Membership criteria were altered to admit physiotherapists in 1958 and to incorporate medical students and physical educators in 1961. Consequently, membership doubled within two years (from 100–200) and rose to 450 in 1968 (Heggie 2011). However, for most of its history BASM would be a representative rather than a regulatory body (Carter 2009b), unable to establish authoritative and definitive status or to effectively police competing occupations. Crucial in this was the competition between various agencies for control of the intersection of sport and medicine, in particular the British Olympic Association (BOA) Medical Committee (est. 1959), and the *Sports Council's* Research and Statistics Committee (1965). Jurisdictional boundary work between these bodies was acrimonious.

The *Sports Council* essentially had a 'community sport' remit but considerable financial resources. Initially it used much of its central government grant to fund research, notably a 1967 research project that somewhat circularly concluded that: (a) sports injuries were distinct because athletes desired to return to competition as quickly as possible; (b) athletes required both early intervention and integrated treatment; and (c) that the demand for and existence of sports medicine bodies/specialists proved that sports injuries were distinct. The *Sports Council* further funded a survey of sports injuries and initiated a 'Sports Injury Clinic Scheme', effectively in an attempt to quantify the scale of the 'problem' and thus justify greater provision. However, the hospital-based methodology employed failed to capture the work of, and thus largely alienated, the majority of BASM members. Whilst these initiatives showed that sports injuries were common amongst the general population and often inadequately treated, they failed to convince government officials that publicly-funded specialist medical treatment was either necessary or a priority (Heggie 2011).

Conversely, the BOA was solely concerned with elite performers yet had relatively limited finance. However, its access to and influence over elite athletes was a key resource and consequently it was the BOA, funded by the Medical Research Council (MRC), which launched the 1965 Mexican Research Project to explore the effects of altitude on athletic performance. The MRC and BOA fell out over the final report, with Dr Lewis Pugh, a leading but non-sport-specialist scientist, criticized for his failure to appreciate the psychological needs and the competition-based sensitivity of sport-related test data (Heggie 2008). This fuelled perceptions that sports medicine serviced specific yet limited populations. The acclimatization camps subsequently organized in Switzerland 'established the BOA's Medical Committee as a permanent and authoritative source of medical advice and guidance' (Heggie 2011: 123).

By contrast, BASM had multiple ad hoc contacts with national governing bodies of sport but neither money nor privileged access. Consequently, BASM mainly existed through arranging lectures and meetings, and providing 'expert advice' about the elite sport population when invited to do so. Some members provided occasional injury clinics but not as recognizably BASM entities. Consequently, it was the *Sports Council* rather than BASM that intervened to mediate between the BBBC and the RCP when the latter wanted to undertake an inquiry into the dangers of boxing (see previous section), and which in 1978 responded on behalf of the Minister for Sport to the Council of Europe's request for information about sports medicine and science in Britain (Heggie 2011). BASM's claims to professional expertise were therefore unconvincing.

Indicative of the acrimonious relations within British sports medicine were the (largely) failed collaborative ventures. The BOA, BASM and Physical Education Association (PEA) cooperated over the 1963 establishment of the Institute of Sports Medicine (ISM) but BASM became aggrieved when the ISM changed its constitution to make BASM's presence by invitation rather than statutory. BASM opposed the ISM's attempts to establish a diploma in 1976, arguing that it was impossible to embrace the multidisciplinarity of sports medicine (in Britain) in a single diploma, and that the European-derived syllabus on which it would be based was inferior to existing British practice (Heggie 2011). BASM also openly criticized the BOA's medical provision at the 1972 Olympics and fell out with the *Sports Council* over the foundation of the London (later National) Sports Medicine Institute in 1986 (Heggie 2011).

Thus, BASM ostensibly became an umbrella body of healthcare professionals, and while medicine was ascendant, other occupations were more effective in establishing their own independent bodies (see Chapter 7 for a discussion of the professionalization of physiotherapy). Consequently, the multidisciplinarity of BASM meant that there was no organization specifically representing sports doctors. Recognition of this led to the creation of the British Association of Trauma in Sport (BATS) in 1980, with membership restricted to registered medical practitioners. However, those who had founded BATS to push harder for specialist status were accused of being self-serving due to their role as advisors to a company providing members with insurance cover (Heggie 2011). Debates about the explicit recognition of doctors within sports medicine continued, with calls for a federated structure for BASM in the 1980s, and the formation of the United Kingdom Association of Doctors in Sports in 2001.

Further restricting BASM's claim for authoritative status in the field was the disaggregation of people providing healthcare for elite athletes. The clearest example relates to 'football club doctors and physiotherapists, who were independent of BAS(E)M [and] felt little loyalty to it or a need to defer to it on medical matters' (Carter 2009b: 71). As the most commercialized sport of the late nineteenth/early twentieth century, football was at the forefront of employing full-time trainers (many referred to as 'physiotherapists' despite a lack of appropriate qualifications), appointing medical officers and was involved in the certification of players' fitness to play. The doctors were largely subordinate to the management and players within the masculine culture of professional football. Indicative of the traditional coupling of vocationalism and professionalism in general practice (Jones and Green 2006), and subscribing to the tradition of voluntarism in British medicine and society (Carter 2012b), their reward was rarely financial; often simply the social prestige of being involved in the local football club (see Chapter 7 for further discussion).

Finally, pioneers of British sports medicine have described resistance from the broader medical profession. During the *Sports Medicine Witness Seminar* (Reynolds and Tansey 2009: 22; 36) Peter Sperryn spoke of the 'vindictive hostility' that created the need to 'fight every inch of the way' to establish the specialism. He recalled being turned down for jobs due to prejudice against sports medicine: 'a very senior censor of the Royal College of Physicians, said: "Ah, sports medicine, what's that? What's in the bucket, a sponge?"' (Reynolds and Tansey 2009: 21). Similarly, John

Lloyd Parry reflected that, 'the initial stumbling block to professional status appears to have been the hostility of the medical establishment and their reluctance to acknowledge the progress of the discipline despite the achievements and demands of sports medicine itself' (Reynolds and Tansey 2009: xxvii).

Thus, British sports medicine was more organic than organized, more pervasive than powerful, and more dispersed than distinctive. What was the catalyst that moved sports medicine from 'Cinderella status ... practised away from mainstream medicine as a hobby or in the domains of private practice and physiotherapy', to a 'single respected voice to coordinate education, research, service provision and accreditation'? (Batt and Macleod 1997: 621).

As in Canada, national governing bodies of sport and government agencies began to bemoan the underdeveloped state of sports medicine in Britain. In 1988, the *Sports Council* argued that, 'the need has never been greater for British sportspeople ... to have access to adequate medical and scientific support when and where they need it' (cited in Green and Houlihan, 2005: 139). Further impetus came through the government's publication of plans to establish an 'academy' to coordinate elite sport development (DNH 1995). In *Sport and Exercise Medicine: Policy and Provision* the BMA (1996) responded to these changes and outlined an agenda for change. The subsequent UK Sports Institute (UKSI) would, according to Minister for Sport, Tony Banks, 'professionalise' UK sport and establish a 'medals factory' (Theodoraki 1999). In 2002 it was restructured as the Home Countries Institutes of Sport (HCIS) and by 2005 Green and Houlihan (2005: 139) would note that, 'an integrated, multi-disciplinary sports science and sports medicine programme is now emerging'. Funding for Summer Olympic sports rose from £70 million in the four years up to 2004 (Athens), to £261 million prior to London 2012 and reached almost £350 million for Rio 2016. It was no coincidence that the decision to recognize sports medicine as a medical speciality in Britain came just a few months before London secured the right to host the 2012 Olympic Games.

But perhaps what is unique about the British development of sports medicine is that the traits of a profession, if it is ever meaningful to reify these as an 'achievement', have been predicated on supplanting a performance-orientation with a public health mission. While a key stimulus for change is the demand for elite sport provision, state mandate was ultimately secured by embracing the physical activity for public health agenda (Batt and Cullen 2005). Indicative of this shift in emphasis is BAS(E)M's changing mission statement. We saw above how initially Adolphe Abrahams made no explicit reference to public health but highlighted instead training and sports injuries. By 2009, the emphasis had been significantly revised such that performance considerations were relegated to the final two words of BASEM's 64-word Mission statement:

The aims of the Association are to promote and study methods for the protection and improvement of public health and fitness amongst members of the public participating in sporting, recreational and other leisure-time activities. BASEM also endeavours to promote research into the causation and treatment of medical problems arising from such activities and into the scientific and psychological aspects of athletic and sporting achievement.

Moreover, by 2015, despite nearly quadrupling the length of the mission statement, BASEM had reconfigured its aims to be entirely focused on promotion of the 'profession' through contributions to the broader social health agenda and the removal of reference to elite sport entirely (see Box 3.3).

Indicative of the ongoing tensions within sports medicine, a National Centre for Sport and Exercise Medicine, established as a 2012 Olympic

---

Box 3.3 The Objectives of BASEM (2015)

1   To promote exercise as a therapeutic tool.
2   To support and promote the multi-disciplinary team in sport and exercise medicine.
3   To support the professional needs of those doctors working in the speciality of sport and exercise medicine and to advise on career structures in sport and exercise medicine.
4   To provide support and education for those healthcare professionals involved in the care of athletes and individuals undertaking, or aspiring to undertake regular physical activity at all levels.
5   To promote the speciality of sport and exercise medicine and to encourage best standards of clinical practice in the care of the exercising individual. To promote the adoption of evidence-based practice in all areas of sport and exercise medicine.
6   To support and encourage research in sport and exercise medicine.
7   To promote the adoption of exercise and physical activity by all sections of the population for their general well-being and in the preventions of illness.
8   To assist and advise all relevant authorities in adopting policies that will encourage and promote physical activity in schools, the work place and the home.
9   To cooperate with the Faculty of Sport and Exercise Medicine and the Institute of Sport and Exercise Medicine and to collaborate with other Associations, both nationally and internationally, in furthering the speciality of sport and exercise medicine and the aims of BASEM.
10 To communicate frequently and effectively with the membership.

Source: www.basem.co.uk/about-us/association-objectives.html. Accessed 24 February 2015.

legacy project, had no connection to, or representation from, BASEM. There is also a disconnect between the public health emphasis of sports medicine policy and what sport and exercise medicine registrars identify as important aspects of their work (O'Halloran *et al.* 2009). Conversely, *Sport and Exercise Medicine: A Fresh Approach* (Jones *et al.* 2011), a document designed to 'introduce SEM [sport and exercise medicine] to the NHS' identified four areas of practice: physical activity in the prevention of disease; physical activity in the treatment of disease; musculoskeletal health; and workplace wellness. It defined sports medicine specialists as trained in chronic disease management, the prescription of exercise, the diagnosis and management of musculoskeletal disorders and the education and training of MDTs. The scope of sports medicine research it identified predominantly related to physical activity interventions. The document contained little mention of sports injuries as distinct and/or requiring specific intervention.

Conclusion

Contrary to the dominant thesis (Hoberman 1992; Waddington 1996) performance is hardly the raison d'être of sports medicine in Britain, if indeed elsewhere. Heggie (2010a: 459) also misrepresents the case claiming that sports medicine 'now extends into community sport and public health'. In Britain, perhaps due to its relatively late formal recognition as a medical speciality, the emergence of a sports medicine specialism has been a direct result of the re-conceptualization of health. In this regard, the development of sports medicine is an institutional manifestation of medicalization at a conceptual level.

However, while sports medicine has undergone many of the processes normally association with professionalization, such is the international and temporal diversity of these developments that it is impossible to write a single or uniform narrative. That sports medicine has been dogged by definitional imprecision is partly a consequence as well as a cause of the speciality's weakness, partly a driving factor behind its interdisciplinarity and partly a result of its failed attempts to convince others of its authoritative status. Similarly, we see representative bodies for sports medicine in contextually specific tensions with other medical groups, with sports organizations and with state authorities. Through the various cases reviewed we see the ebb and flow of medicalization and processes that empower non-medical or para-medical groups; advances on some fronts, accompanied by regressions on others.

Despite this, two common themes emerge. While a health rationale has frequently been necessary to legitimize the specialism, in many cases performance has provided additional weight to convince others to accept and fund sports medicine. Moreover, while the nature of sports performance has certainly changed during the twentieth century, the *notion* of health has perhaps changed more fundamentally (see Chapter 2). The failure to justify the formalization of Canadian sports medicine on public health grounds in the 1950s compares strikingly with the decisive role health has played in the development of British sports medicine in the early twenty-first century.

Second, part historical legacy and part contributory factor to these professional developments, is the relative independence of sports medicine. If sports medicine has partly been defined by the performance orientation of sport, so it has also been shaped by the semi-autonomy of what Bourdieu might call the sport field (evident, for example, in the longstanding commitment to amateurism, the internal regulation of violence that would in other contexts be criminalized, and even the sport–health ideology). As we have seen, sports medicine has frequently stood at a distance from and in dispute with 'mainstream' medicine. This has been both imposed upon (i.e. the development of sex testing and policing the health of boxers), and driven by (i.e. in making the case for a distinctive area of practice) sports medicine, itself 'structurally and culturally distinct' from 'mainstream' medicine (Malcolm 2006a). We explore these dimensions further in Chapters 7 and 8 but first we explore how the sports-related institutional manifestations of medicalization have intersected with the re-conceptualization of health outlined in Chapter 2 and how that is evident in the recent growth of PAHP policies.

Chapter 4

Sport, medicine and public health

As illustrated in Chapter 1, in recent years there has been an explosion in the number and frequency of health promotion campaigns that feature sport, exercise and physical activity. Physical activity health promotion (PAHP) has not just joined alcohol, tobacco and diet to become one of the four main targets of health promotion, but is claimed to be 'today's best buy in public health' (AMRC 2015; DoH 2009a). These policies are premised on and serve to perpetuate the enduring sport–health ideology, but their contemporary manifestation is also inextricably tied to the development of what Armstrong (1995) termed surveillance medicine, the reconceptualization of health identified by Crawford (2006) and others, and the development of NPH (Lupton 1995). Fundamentally, moreover, they also represent a key stage in the medicalization of sport and the professional project of sports medicine.

This chapter extends these introductory comments through an examination of the role of sport, exercise and physical activity in contemporary health promotion campaigns. It builds on existing critiques of health promotion per se, and PAHP in particular. While it concludes by examining comparable developments in America, the bulk of the analysis in this chapter focuses on nine PAHP documents published in the UK since 2004. These are:

> *At Least Five a Week: Evidence of the Impact of Physical Activity and its Relationship With Health* (DoH 2004);
> *Be Active, be Healthy* (DoH 2009a);
> *Let's get Moving* (DoH 2009b);
> *Exercise for Life: Physical Activity in Health and Disease* (RCP 2012);
> *Moving More, Living More. The Physical Activity Olympic and Paralympic Legacy for the Nation* (HM Govt and Mayor of London 2014);
> *Turning the Tide of Inactivity* (UKactive 2014);
> *Everybody Active, Everyday: An Evidence Based Approach to Physical Activity* (PHE 2014);

Tackling Physical Activity – A Coordinated Approach (APCPA 2014); and
Exercise: The Miracle Cure and the Role of the Doctor in Promoting it (AMRC 2015).

By undertaking a developmental approach we not only see the similarities and differences between PAHP and other forms of health promotion, but reveal the underlying process of knowledge production. The overriding trope of the last decade has been for policy to shift from trying to establish the case for the health promoting benefits of exercise (DoH 2004) to positioning exercise as 'a miracle cure ... if physical activity were a drug it would be classed as a wonder drug' (AMRC 2015: 2). The outcome has not (solely) been a consequence of the persuasiveness of the evidence, but also as a consequence of broader social processes that have seen the alignment of diverse interest groups. Ultimately this analysis illustrates how, specifically at a conceptual level, PAHP is a consequence of and has contributed to the medicalization of sport.

The sociology of public health promotion

As public health campaigns have extended the process of medicalization so sociological critiques of their form and impact have developed. These critiques tend to focus on three interrelated issues: *structure, surveillance* and *consumption* (Nettleton and Bunton 1995). *Structurally*, health promotion can be criticized for failing to recognize the importance of material (dis-) advantage in mediating lifestyle and disregarding the living conditions of relative poverty in contouring the choices that people can make. Such policies frequently exhibit 'lifestyle drift', or 'a tendency for policy to start off recognising the need for action on upstream social determinants of health inequalities only to drift downstream to focus largely on individual lifestyle factors' (Popay *et al.* 2010: 148). Evidence suggests that health promotion aimed at individual behavioural change is most effective in relation to populations in favourable social and economic conditions and thus campaigns frequently perpetuate inequalities (Baum and Fisher 2014). Moreover, the dominance of psychological paradigms in health promotion leads to an advocacy of individual responsibility for health (Horrocks and Johnson 2014), and consequently such policies facilitate victim-blaming and stigmatization.

Health promotion has also been criticized for monitoring and regulating populations through *surveillance*. The NPH falsely depicts the 'unhealthy' as 'abnormal' when, according to the assessment tools designed by health promoters themselves, they exhibit common and therefore essentially normal behaviour. Consequently, the population becomes 'profiled' into distinct and hierarchically ranked social groups with those who are successful or competent self-managers of health viewed as virtuous (Timmermans 2013). Because healthy living becomes not something one merely does, but part of a broader personal philosophy of continuous self-improvement, health promotion enables medicine to extend its reach beyond the impact that consulting doctors alone could ever achieve. The reach and extent of surveillance is evidenced by the construction of new social identities, as described in the notion of healthism (Crawford 2006).

Finally, it is argued that health promotion blurs the boundaries between medicine and consumer culture in adopting the techniques of commercial marketing, and creating distinct and socially desirable lifestyles, which in turn reinforce social stratification. An adjunct to the belief that health status is transposed onto the body is the reality that certain (higher status) social groups are better placed to attain said body through engagement with the marketplace. For instance, Jennifer Smith-Maguire (2008) uses the phrase 'fit for consumption, fit to be consumed', to illustrate in a Bourdieuian sense the interdependence of physical and economic capital. Specifically, the wealthier (and therefore those with longer and higher quality life expectancy) are better able to join gyms, etc., and so become increasingly healthy, which contributes to greater physical capital, which in turn helps generate greater wealth. It is for this reason that studies consistently show a high correlation between social capital and physical activity levels (Legh-Jones and Moore 2012). Indeed Pampel's (2012: 397) analysis shows a stronger statistical correlation between reading and BMI than between exercise and BMI, suggesting that, 'the physical nature of leisure-time activity may be less important [in determining BMI] than its cultural meaning'.

The work of Deborah Lupton (1995) is perhaps the most prominent of the critiques of the contemporary manifestations of public health. Lupton identifies a range of inherent contradictions and (un-)intended and iatrogenic consequences which stem from NPH policies. For example, NPH implies that the state will provide for people's needs, but then tells people what those needs are; it assumes that citizens are at once rational consumers but also misguided in their current choices; it is premised on empowerment yet serves largely to perpetuate the dominance of experts. NPH represents an extension of the medicalization process in the sense of both defining social problems and locating medicine as fundamental to their resolution.

Lupton (1995: 49) highlights the importance of the process of knowledge production that underpins health promotion, arguing for 'an explicit questioning of whose voices are being heard and privileged, the alliances and conflicts involved, what body of expertise is cited in support, "what counts as knowledge", how it is organized, controlled, authenticated and disseminated'. NPH relies on epidemiology which, beyond simply discovering the causes of disease, has a number of broader social consequences

(Petersen and Lupton 1996). Epidemiology depends upon and so justifies the routine monitoring of populations. It isolates risk variables and places them in a hierarchy, which tends to emphasize individual responsibility and diminish the role of social structural factors. Attempts to quantify essentially qualitative data exaggerate the predictive power of this approach, and while this imprecision is routinely recognized by epidemiologists themselves, it does not radically undermine the dominance of this approach. Any lingering uncertainty is lost or obscured in state and media uses of epidemiological data. Epidemiology persists despite what has been termed the 'prevention paradox'; i.e. that proscribed behaviour may bring 'much benefit to the population, but offers little to each participating individual' (Rose 1981, cited in Kreiner and Hunt 2013). Moreover, the approach favours the measurement of certain outputs (e.g. time-limited behavioural, rather than long-term social structural, change) and concomitantly overlooks the lived experience of health/illness. Evidence of the failure of behavioural change interventions rarely informs subsequent policy (Baum and Fisher 2014). Crucially, 'the very choice of what phenomena require measurement and surveillance is a product of sociocultural processes' including the interests of individual researchers and their employers, the relative ease of measurement and the broader political priorities for research funding (Petersen and Lupton 1996: 36). Thus, epidemiology largely monitors numerically limited and easily accessed populations such as those participating in physical activity interventions, and neglects diverse, dispersed or isolated individuals, including those with SRI.

A critique of physical activity health promotion

The critiques of surveillance and structure are particularly applicable to PAHP. Compared with the other main targets of health promotion, a distinct feature of PAHP is that desirable levels of activity are relatively elusive which, in turn, emphasizes the importance of continuous self-improvement. While PAHP documents have, for 20 years, consistently proscribed that adults should undertake 30 minutes of moderate intensity exercise five times a week, with moderate intensity defined as making an individual 'slightly out of breath' (e.g. ACSM 1990; AMRC 2015), in comparison with the person who smokes 0 cigarettes or consumes fewer than 14 units of alcohol per week, the goals of PAHP are both more subjective (what is *slight* breathlessness?) and more dynamic (the exertion required to invoke breathlessness will increase as one exercises more regularly). This is compounded by the fact that whereas other health promotion campaigns largely focus on persuading the public to *reduce* their consumption (dietary campaigns urging people to consume at least five portions of fruit/vegetables a day are an exception), PAHP emphasizes *increased* exercise participation with a subtext of 'more is better'. This is explicit in the title of *At Least Five a Week* (DoH 2004) and the text of *Exercise for Life*, which states that healthcare professionals 'should always look to advise patients to increase their levels of physical activity' (RCP 2012: 5). *Everybody Active, Everyday* (PHE 2014) advocates an engagement which, if taken literally, will redefine a person's life and, inevitably, sense of self. Thus, compared with smokers and alcohol drinkers in particular, the exerciser's happiness and healthiness are imprecisely defined, elusive and therefore relatively unobtainable goals. PAHP epitomizes the way in which NPH invokes population surveillance with goals that encourage citizens to voluntarily and continuously compel themselves to self-manage health and in so doing redefine identity through lifestyle (Lupton 1995).

A further characteristic of these policies is the way in which concerns about the social structural determinants of health become obscured by the emphasis on individualistic behavioural change. *At Least Five a Week* (DoH 2004: iii) presents the goal of increasing physical activity levels as complex – 'a tremendous public health challenge' – and requiring a 'cultural shift' which focuses on both personal attitudes and structural/environmental issues. But while policies continue to recognize that physical activity patterns are significantly influenced by ethnicity and household income (DoH 2009a), gender and disability (HM Govt and Mayor of London 2014), economic deprivation and the poor provision of leisure facilities (UKactive 2014) – indeed seven of the nine legally protected equalities in the UK (age, disability, economic, gender identity, geographic, race, and sexual orientation) (PHE 2014) – they exhibit 'lifestyle drift' (Popay *et al.* 2010) in their reduction of such complexity to one 'simple answer to many of the big health challenges' (DoH 2009b: 8), i.e. active lifestyles. Indicatively, 'what we need to do is simple: move more' (APCPA 2014: 5). However, the notion that 'we all need to do more' (DoH 2009b: 6) essentially locates the solution with the individual.

In envisaging that such policies will effectively 'enable people to take control' (PHE 2014: 4), PAHP perpetuates the promise of empowerment that characterizes health promotion (NB: *Turning the Tide* (UKactive 2014) is an exception in that it specifically focuses on action to be taken by the government, local authorities and activity sector). The hypothetical examples presented in *Exercise: The Miracle Cure* (AMRC 2015), both illustrate this point and provide an example of victim-blaming through such individualization. In one scenario two office workers – Angela and Tracy – present to their GP with raised blood pressure, mild depression and back pain. The GP advises them both to be more active and avoid long periods sitting. Angela, joins a cycle-to-work scheme and lowers her blood pressure, loses weight, relieves her back pain and starts cycling with her son at weekends. Conversely, Tracy does not change her behaviour, her back pain worsens, she takes medication for her blood pressure which makes her drowsy, she falls off her mobility scooter fracturing her humerus (weakened by inactivity-induced osteoporosis), and becomes unemployed following surgery and extensive physiotherapy treatment. The structural conditions (Angela's supporting employer) are lost amidst a narrative whereby individual agency directly equates with personal health and happiness. Stigmatization is inherent.

Given the alarmist and rather evangelical tenor of (some) PAHP, one might assume that evidence for its efficacy was incontrovertible. Yet as noted, NPH is itself a product of its social context; of the changing disease burden and economic exigencies (Nettleton 2006). Moreover, as previous critiques of PAHP policies have identified, the underlying science is far less objective or conclusive than frequently portrayed. For instance, Bercovitz (2000) argues that the 'Active Living' campaign implemented in Canada in the 1990s should be understood in relation to a broader socio-economic-political-historical context including the Ben Johnson drugs scandal (which undermined the hegemony of performance sport in Canada), and the rise of a neo-liberal political agenda to reduce state expenditure and healthcare costs. Pointing to the variance of physical activity scales, definitional inconsistencies and recruitment problems which lead to sample bias, Bercovitz (2000: 26) argues that the underlying science is a 'political and ideological' construct. Similarly, Piggin and Bairner (2016) highlight how the medical community plays a fundamental role in legitimizing 'scientific facts' which come to constitute knowledge about physical activity. In a critique of a *Lancet* (2012) special issue focusing on a global physical inactivity pandemic, Piggin and Bairner highlight contradictory claims about: the existing knowledge of the relationship between physical activity and health (e.g. 'centuries old' and 'just emerging'); a failure to engage with evidence from social scientific research which would temper inflated claims about Olympic physical activity legacies; and the use of nostalgia as a rhetorical technique to reconstruct the history of physical activity and health promotion (see also Smith and Green 2006). The authors conclude that, 'the complexities inherent within the global pandemic metanarrative disrupt the possibility of rigorous argument' (Piggin and Bairner 2016: 143).

As useful as these critiques are, a focus on individual policies essentially provides a snapshot rather than a holistic understanding of these processes. In seeking to understand the medicalization of sport it is important to ask not simply what are the impacts of PAHP, or what evidence there is for such impacts, but how they have come to be so socially pervasive? Thus, in the following sections we undertake a developmental and comparative analysis of the production of knowledge underpinning UK PAHP policy documents. First however, because it is fundamental to the subsequent critique, we take a brief detour to explore the epidemiology of SRI.

The injury impact of sport/exercise: epidemiological evidence

The problems of accurately harvesting SRI data are widely recognized. As we saw in Chapter 3, sports medicine's historical struggle to be identified as a discrete area of practice stems from the inability to delineate aspects of its practice (e.g. treating sports injuries) relative to other areas of medicine. Indeed, the International Classification of Diseases reflects this, providing no category that is either all-embracing, or exclusive to SRI (Kisser and Bauer 2012). Quantification problems are subsequently compounded by the non-standardized definitions employed in studies (e.g. 'sport', 'exercise' and/or 'recreation' injuries) and the demographics of the population surveyed (younger and male cohorts consistently return the highest rates of SRI). The way injury is defined (e.g. requiring medical consultation, work absenteeism, or cessation of sport/exercise) is also important. There is, further, no standard way to contextualise findings and consequently SRI data may, for example, be presented as a proportion of all injuries/medical visits, per head of population, per sports participant or per sporting hour/week/year (Pollock 2014). As indicated in Chapter 1, different activities have very different injury rates. Seasonal and cross-cultural differences in sports participation make international comparisons more problematic. While a previous overview of the costs of SRIs concluded that epidemiological information is incomplete and inconsistent, it went on to say that data were 'interesting, if sometimes alarming', and merit further attention (White 2004: 308).

One response is, like Petersen and Lupton (1996), to disregard epidemiology in its entirety and its data as social fabrication. However, this position falsely homogenizes the epidemiological community for, in reality, epidemiologists themselves forward different agendas. Rather more interesting, and notwithstanding the methodological difficulties, analysis of the SRI epidemiology literature reveals the underlying knowledge production process. What follows is, by necessity, an overview of estimates of: (a) the prevalence of SRI; and (b) their social impact. Unequivocally though, it demonstrates that the number of SRI is significant both in itself and relative to the broader social health burden and thus it fundamentally problematizes some of the claims of PAHP.

The prevalence of sport-related injury

Because of the relative ease with which data can be collected, many epidemiological studies of SRI are based around emergency medicine (EM) consultations. The problems of this, however, are illustrated by UK government data in which the reason for attendance in 95% of cases is essentially unclassified (4.8% not known, 90.4% 'other'). Of the remaining 4.8%, 'sport injury' is the largest single category of cases (1.9%), above road accidents (1.4%), assaults (0.8%) and deliberate self-harm (0.6%). Illustrative of the complexity of categorization, the two largest sub-categories of road accidents (pedal cyclist in non-collision transport accidents (17.5%) and pedestrians injured by a car (11.8%)) involve people behaving in accordance with PAHP advice (HSCIC 2014a).

Studies that specifically assess the impact of SRIs in EM promise greater specificity but are plagued by inconsistencies. Sandelin *et al.* (1985), Hockey and Knowles (2000), and Kisser and Bauer (2012) estimate that sports injuries account for a significant proportion of *acute injuries* presented to EM (up to 14%), while studies that locate SRIs as a proportion of *all* EM consultations provide estimates from 9% (de Loes 1990) to 3.6% (Bedford and MacAuley 1984; see also Abernethy *et al.* 2002; Jones and Taggart 1994; Murphy *et al.* 1992; Watters *et al.* 1984). One explanation for this variance is the definitional categories employed (e.g. 'sport' as opposed to 'sport and recreation injuries'), timing of study and the age profile of the sample. For example, 'sport and recreational injuries' have been shown to account for up to 28% of EM visits made by children (Sceats and Gilles 1989; Burt and Overpeck 2001).

However, in many respects SRIs treated in EM represent the tip of the iceberg (Boyce and Quigley 2004) because 'many sports injuries are chronic or overuse in nature and are consequently unlikely to be treated in hospital' (Finch and Kenihan 2001). Cassell *et al.* (2003) estimate the ratio of hospital admissions, EM visits and GP consultations to be 1:11:12. Similarly Baarveld *et al.* (2011) claim that approximately 50% of SRIs are presented to a family practitioner, while Mummery *et al.* (2002) estimate that 11% are presented to EM, 31.4% to a GP, and 22.1% to a physiotherapist. As with medicine in general, evidence suggests that this process is gendered with females particularly likely to seek chiropractice, osteopathy, acupuncture and physiotherapy treatment rather than attend EM (Mitchell *et al.* 2010). Research on attendance at sports injury clinics suggests that for over 60% this is their first engagement with medical practitioners (Rowell and Rees-Jones 1988).

Population studies provide a similarly diverse range of estimates. The proportion found to have experienced SRIs in the previous year varies: 3.1% in Germany (Schneider *et al.* 2006), 5.9% in Australia (Egger 1991), 7.4% in Ontario (McClaren 1996), 10.1% in Canada (McCutcheon *et al.* 1997), 16.6% in Queensland (Mummery *et al.* 2002) and 18% in the Netherlands (van der Sluis *et al.* 1998). A study of the adult population in England and Wales reported that 8.1% incurred a SRI in the four weeks prior to survey, which equated to 18% of the sports-active population (Nicholl *et al.* 1995). On this basis Nicholl *et al.* estimate that there are 19.3 million new sports injuries a year in England and Wales, plus 10.4 million recurrent injuries, making a total of 29.7 million SRIs per year in England and Wales.

The impact of sport-related injury

While population studies further indicate that the majority of SRIs are never medically treated (just 43% according to van Mechelen *et al.* 1992), it would be false to assume from this that they tend not to be serious. While there is a perception that the relative triviality of SRIs is evidenced by the frequent lack of medical consultation, it has also been argued that lack of access, expected length of wait, perceived lack of expertise in primary care, and prevailing perceptions that such injuries are self-inflicted (and therefore less 'worthy' of treatment) dissuade people from presenting SRIs to medical personnel (Knill-Jones 1997, see Chapter 5 for an illustration). Despite this, Nicholl *et al.* (1995) estimate that over half the 19.3 million new SRIs in England and Wales each year were 'potentially serious' (e.g. fractures, dislocations, head injuries), required medical assistance or restricted normal activities. Moreover, it should be noted that Kisser and Bauer (2012) estimate that there are more deaths in the 27 EU member states due to sports participation (7000 per year) than to workplace accidents (6080) or homicides (5540). Mueller *et al.* (1996) state that 7% of all para- and quadriplegia injuries are sport-related and that 10% of all brain injuries are a result of 'sport or recreation' (the latter very likely to be an underestimate, see Chapter 9). Dekker (2003a) found that 32% of those who took time off work due to a sports injury continued to experience problems for an average of 2.8 years after the initial incident. Finally Burt and Overpeck (2001) argue that, according to a variety of measures – treatment, costs, time – SRIs are equal in severity to non-SRIs presented to EM.

Attempts to put a financial cost to this health burden (e.g. Dekker *et al.* 2003a, 2003b; van Mechelen *et al.* 1992) normally categorize costs as direct (medical), indirect (e.g. through loss of work) and social (e.g. quality of life), enabling both a comparison of direct and indirect costs of different types of injury and, in some cases, an explicit cost-benefit assessment of SRI and inactivity. The former consistently estimate direct costs of SRI as constituting only a relatively minor proportion of overall cost. For instance, a Canadian government survey (1998/1999) estimated that direct costs accounted for 36.2% (cited in White 2004), while Nicholl *et al.* (1995) found that direct treatment of new and recurrent injuries constituted 42.3% of total costs. Factoring in social costs is perhaps more speculative but closer to the real overall cost. Weaver *et al.*'s (1999) study of high school SRIs (and thus a younger cohort) estimated that direct medical costs equated to 6.5% of the total, while Finch *et al.* (2001) claim that across the adult population social costs account for 81% of total SRI costs.

Cost-benefit analyses, however, most directly problematize the rationale for PAHP. Kisser and Bauer's (2012) analysis of Swiss and Austrian data found that the health costs of treating SRIs accounted for 41% and 53% of estimated health savings of physical activity respectively. Similarly, Nicholl *et al.* (1995) estimate that the state annually spent £420 million on the medical treatment of SRIs which, *without* adjusting for inflation, represented approximately 40% of the estimated direct cost of physical inactivity in the UK a decade later (Allender *et al.* 2007; DoH 2004; Scarborough *et al.* 2011). This study further explored the cost-benefit for different age groups and concluded that sports participation for younger adults (15–44) entailed a net cost of £25 per person, and a net benefit of £20 per person for those over 45 (Nicholl *et al.* 1994). Others have noted that the health burdens are not only stratified according to age and type of sport, but also by participants' gender and social class (Pollock and Kirkwood 2008).

Given the aforementioned methodological concerns, the aim has not been to provide a definitive statement about the incidence and impact of SRIs. To reiterate, we currently have:

> incomplete knowledge about the size of the public health sports injury burden, very little evidence about the existence of effective prevention solutions, a total lack of implementation activities across the population and no information at all about cost-effectiveness or cost-benefit scenarios associated with investments in the interventions at the population level.
>
> (Finch 2012: 73)

Moreover, a comparison of the cost of population-wide physical inactivity with SRI costs of a necessarily limited and difficult to define population is fraught with complications. For instance, while 67% of men and 55% of women self-report meeting the recommendations for aerobic activity, objective measures show that just 6% of men and 4% of women actually do (HSCIC 2014b). Furthermore can we assume that, if the 15.3 million adults in England believed to play sport at least once a week were to double, SRI costs would increase proportionately? Simply stated, we do not know the potential costs of PAHP because we do not know how many people this will effect, what activities they might adopt, and with what resultant rate of injury. However, what this section does clearly demonstrate is that participation in sport, exercise and physical activity entails a health cost and that those costs are at least *not* negligible and potentially greater than the savings resulting from increased physical activity. The importance of this conclusion becomes increasingly apparent as we explore the knowledge production process underlying PAHP documents.

Physical activity health promotion and knowledge production

As noted previously, critiques of the sport–health ideology have long charted the tendency for public health policies to conflate sport and exercise despite their distinct health outcomes (Scambler 2005; Waddington 2000). However, a notable feature of UK policies of the last decade has been the addition of physical activity into this elision. The latter has been specifically invoked to embrace activities such as heavy housework and manual work (PHE 2014), gardening, dancing and playing as a family (DoH 2009a) as health enhancing. In part, this change has come through: (a) recognition that sports participation is viewed as particularly unappealing to some sectors of society; (b) the belief that significant health gains can be achieved by relatively minor changes in activity levels; and (c) (somewhat sceptically perhaps) the desire to identify more achievable targets. However, the physical activity agenda remains firmly attached to the sporting sphere. For instance, in *Be Active, be Healthy* (DoH 2009a: 7), the government sought to 'retain and resource those elements of the existing delivery network that can contribute to the wider delivery of physical activity and remain fully aligned with the delivery of sport'.

Such changes in emphasis are often socio-politically driven (Bercovitz 2000). Notably, while the reports published by medical organizations primarily refer to exercise (AMRC 2015; RCP 2012), those published by more overtly political bodies consistently and exclusively refer to activity. Ironically though, it is the latter that make the most frequent and explicit link to sport. Publications prior to London's hosting of the 2012 Olympic and Paralympic Games consistently referred to the potential to 'inspire a generation' (DoH 2009a, 2009b), while in launching *Moving More* (HM Govt. and Mayor of London 2014) Prime Minister David Cameron spoke of the 'need to build ... [on] the spirit of the games ... sport heroes and their many achievements ... creating a nation that's physically active and improving health for the long term'. The bias is replicated in the visual images employed. For instance, 11 of the 12 pictures contained in *Tackling Physical Inactivity* (APCPA 2014) feature people taking part in sports, and seven of those are team sports. Conversely, PAHP documents contain few images of gardening, housework, etc. Commitment to the sport–health ideology leads sport to be used as a tool to inspire and evoke change, while the explicit focus on physical activity stems from an implicit recognition of the epidemiological findings that less intensive exercise has a better cost-benefit heath return. Definitional fluidity enables the emphasis of supportive findings and the concomitant marginalization of problematic epidemiological data.

This point is underscored by changes over time in the way PAHP documents treat the potential health costs of sport and exercise (and physical activity). *At least* (DoH 2004) explicitly sought to assess the 'scientific evidence on the links between physical activity and health' and concluded that the health savings of increased physical activity are 'compelling'. However, the report also includes a 6-page discussion of the 'risks of physical activity', which identifies 'injury as a potential downside of participation' (DoH 2004: 73). Citing the usual methodological caveats, the report notes that the greatest risks are faced by those who do vigorous or 'excessive' amounts of exercise, and those who have, or are at high risk of developing, musculoskeletal disease. It reports Nicholl *et al*.'s (1995) estimate that SRIs in England and Wales cost £991 million per year (42.3% of which are direct costs) but claimed that 'many' such injuries were avoidable.

Subsequent PAHP documentation disregards the potential health costs of increased physical activity. For instance, *Let's get Moving* (DoH 2009b) makes no mention of sports injuries in an appendix on 'cost implications', and foreclosed any cost-benefit analysis with the claim that the 'cost of inactivity ... is irrefutable' (DoH 2009b). Similarly, *Turning the Tide* (UKactive 2014) identifies development and implementation costs as the only potential 'spend' implications of PAHP programmes, and *Moving More* (HM Govt and Mayor of London 2014) provides a list of economic benefits of physical activity but no consideration of costs. *Exercise* (AMRC 2015) simply states that there is a 'very low risk of injury' from engaging in 'health promoting activity'; a statement which, the epidemiological literature shows, could only be true if activity was narrowly defined to exclude (certain types of) sport and exercise which, of course, no policy has ever suggested it should be.

This change in emphasis is starkly illustrated in a comparison of two reports produced by the Royal College of Physicians: *Medical Aspects of Exercise: Benefits and Risks* (RCP 1991); and *Exercise for Life* (RCP 2012). In addition to the titular reference, the earlier report notes that 'regular physical exercise is not without its own hazards' (RCP 1991: vii) and lists the following examples: cardiac risks; exercise induced asthma; viral infections; haemoglobinuria (damage to red blood cells) and haemorrhage; musculo-skeletal risks; reproductive harm (menstrual dysfunction and subfertility); loss of temperature control; bowel disturbance. However, the introduction to the 2012 report explicitly notes the committee's decision *not* to update the original publication, choosing instead to explore 'issues surrounding the use of exercise in the prevention and management of disease, and ... the barriers to exercise prescription'. It subsequently states the widely held view that 'the risks of exercise are not clear', but provides an unsubstantiated and more problematic extrapolation that 'therefore [they] tend to be overestimated' (RCP 2012: 6).

Finally, the most recent documents have moved full circle in their proposed frameworks for the assessment of PAHP initiatives. Crucially, they all present SRI as an irrelevance and advocate measuring policy impact *solely* in terms of increased activity levels (APCPA 2014; PHE 2014). The process, moreover, concludes with ironic circularity as understanding of the efficacy of physical activity comes to reflect the earlier uncertainty about the impact of SRI. Thus, *Everybody Active, Everyday* (PHE 2014) points to the challenges of ascertaining activity levels in young people, and the need to raise the quality of evidence relating to the impact and investment return of PAHP, *Tackling Physical Inactivity* (APCPA 2014: 15) identifies 'significant limitations to our ability to measure levels of activity' and/or the effectiveness of specific interventions, and *Turning the Tide of Inactivity* (UKactive 2014: 12) states that 'significant improvements need to be made to the collation, coordination and breadth of data'. Paradoxically, therefore, these statements place knowledge about the efficacy and impact of PAHP on a footing akin to our knowledge of SRI. Tellingly though, each of these comments forms part of a call for increased government support for PAHP, and none suggest, to paraphrase the RCP (2012), that existing evaluations tend to be overestimated.

Thus, in the last decade, publications have shifted from estimating, to disregarding, to denying, to proposing evaluative frameworks that will systematically exclude the cost of SRI from the evaluation of PAHP programmes. As Finch (2012) has argued, government departments tend to be uninterested in injuries that only impact on sports participation because they do not translate to an observable and easily measurable cost. This movement not only favours the measurement of outputs that are relatively easy to quantify (Petersen and Lupton 1996), but also those that will not capture the *un*intended impacts of policy implementation. The epidemiological agenda therefore comes to serve the neoliberal political interests. The knowledge that will in future be assembled cannot critically assess or evaluate PAHP, merely provide evidence that either shows policy to be working or suggests that implementation needs to become more effective.

Physical activity health promotion: interdependence and agendas

This process of knowledge production, and the concomitant increased prominence of PAHP, is a consequence of the convergence of a number of broader social processes and interest groups. Increased physical activity has become positioned as a 'miracle cure' because it is seen as either a relatively inexpensive alternative to medical treatment or, more accurately, as a way of displacing health costs from the state to the individual. The neoliberal imperative to reduce the size and cost of the state is particularly evident in *Moving More*, for while the broader narrative proposes that increased physical activity will counter increasing health costs, the accounting more specifically belies the intention to reposition those costs onto the individual. For example, *Moving More* states that promoting cycling and walking is a 'cheap, convenient and easy way to introduce a level of physical activity' (HM Govt and Mayor of London 2014: 13). However, one reason cited for encouraging more people to walk through towns is pedestrians' relatively high commercial spend (estimated to be £147 per person per month more than car drivers). The report further argues that an eight-fold increase in cycling would save the NHS £17 billion over 20 years. However, in simultaneously noting that UK citizens currently spend £2.5 billion per year on cycling, the NHS savings envisioned from this increase in cycling would simultaneously entail individuals spending £400 billion (£2.5 billion $\times 8 \times 20$) or 2350% more!

But beyond the political sphere a particular set of 'alliances and conflicts' (Lupton 1995) exist, which mean that PAHP encounters minimal social resistance. Whereas it has become increasingly evident that big businesses 'invest directly in research and lobbying ... [to support] policies that do not threaten their interests' (Baum and Fisher 2014: 219), PAHP directly *aligns with* rather than against the interests of multinational corporations. Perhaps the most significant convergence of interests in the PAHP sector however is illustrated by the Nike-commissioned *Designed to Move* (DtM) report (Nike 2012). This report is notable for more than doubling previous estimates of the costs of inactivity in the UK at £20 billion (interestingly this figure is prominent in government PAHP documents but ignored in those of medical organizations (AMRC 2015; RCP 2012)). Moreover, despite DtM presenting evidence that identifies workplaces as the major loci for the reduction in physical activity in recent years, leisure habits are targeted as the solution. In so doing, Nike promotes behavioural change which closely aligns with its own commercial interests (Piggin 2014). Part of the appeal of PAHP to governments, therefore, is that it obviates the politically more problematic task of regulating tobacco, alcohol and food manufacturers, which are fundamental to other forms of health promotion (e.g. controlling advertising/packaging, regulating production, or imposing taxes to provide price disincentives).

But most significant of all, perhaps, is the relationship between PAHP and the sports medicine profession. As we saw in Chapter 3, for many years sports medicine struggled to gain formal recognition or professional status. In particular, attempts to chart the incidence of SRI continually failed to make a conclusive case for recognition as a specialism. Through PAHP, sports medicine has not only received an opportunity to forward a professional project, but has seen previous obstacles disappear. Consider the RCP's 2012 report, which was supported by the FSEM, the Faculty of Public Health and Royal College of General Practitioners. The working party assembled further entailed a 'multidisciplinary consultation' with organizations including: the Fitness Industry Association; Physical Activity Alliance; Register of Exercise Professionals; and DoH Physical Activity

Group (RCP 2012). These groups have now come together in a way that contrasts markedly with the history of tensions and conflict in British sports medicine.

This altered configuration has had a transformative impact on both sports medicine and the interdependence of sport and medicine. The calls to 'co-ordinate the efforts of medical and allied health professionals' (RCP 2012: 16) provide explicit evidence of the medicalization of sport. The RCP report argues that medical professionals can contribute to physical-activity-related health benefits by prescribing exercise to manage illness and injury and by raising overall participation rates and 'hence reducing disease' (RCP 2012: 2). It makes the case for the expansion of SEM consultant posts in the NHS claiming that 'the general population must have access to the best specialist advice on exercise for the prevention of illness, for the management of injuries sustained during exercise and the prescription of exercise to treat illness and injury' (RCP 2012: 6). It further outlines the 'need for increased medical engagement in the delivery of exercise in injury and illness', points to 'a lack of leadership and coordination' for prescription exercise and identifies the 'need ... [for] a concerted effort directed at improving medical knowledge and engagement in the process' (RCP 2012: v). However, it explicitly blames the past failure on medicine's lack of confidence in exercise referral schemes due to uncertainty about professional standards in the leisure industry (RCP 2012: 8). The suggested solution lies in the medicalization of the fitness industry, and specifically the statutory regulation of exercise therapists through registration with the Health Professions Council, 'in order to standardise training, maintain standards, and reassure healthcare professionals of their competence' (RCP 2012: 17).

It is clear who the authors feel should preside over this increasingly interdependent relationship, for they claim to have 'identified a need for the medical profession to take a more active lead on physical activity initiatives' (RCP 2012: 15) and concomitantly recommend 'a medically driven national strategy to use exercise in the prevention *and* treatment of disease' (RCP 2012: 16, emphasis in original). Cognisant perhaps of the radical nature of this change, the report explicitly considers the issue of medicalization. In marked contrast to existing histories of sports medicine in Britain, the report states that the limited engagement of the medical profession with sport and exercise in the past was due to a desire to avoid 'medicalising the issue' (RCP 2012: 3). This risk, however, is now described as 'unfounded' because those who would most benefit from this initiative should do so under medical guidance while 'the healthy population welcome advice from their doctors on issues of "wellness"' (RCP 2012: vi). This form of medicalization has thus become central to the professional project of sports medicine. It is explicitly imperialistic and aspires to operate at the conceptual, institutional and individual levels.

Exercise is medicine

While the focus here has been on developments in the UK, they are global in scope. In many ways the policy documents analysed have been inspired by the aforementioned EiM movement (see Chapter 1). Like the PAHP policies discussed, EiM forms an alliance with corporate vested interests – listing *Anytime Fitness* (gym franchise), *Technogym* (manufacturers of gym equipment), *United Health Foundation* (a not-for-profit arm of the United Health Group, the largest providers of private health in the world), *Optum* (suppliers of information and technology-enabled healthcare services), and *Coca-Cola* amongst its global partners – and is premised on accounting that favours moving the economic burden of healthcare onto the individual (Malcolm and Pullen forthcoming). Moreover, in explicitly suggesting that exercise and medicine have (or should) in some sense become synonymous, and advocating the 'prescription' of 'medicine' to entire populations, EiM contributes to the blurring of the health–illness distinction by converging the lived experience of being either well or unwell (Aronowitz 2009). Indeed, EiM represents medicalization in most of the multiple senses in which sociologists use the term. For instance, EiM represents an attempt to redefine a previously unexceptional aspect of social life as medically essential. It threatens to subsume historically significant motivational drives for sports participation – e.g. risk taking, emotional stimulation, the quest for excitement (Elias and Dunning 1986) – under the goals of health and encourages the evaluation of health outcomes through the use of technology such as heart rate monitors. Despite couching this development within an emphasis on social and lifestyle factors, the EiM initiative effectively expands the role, and consolidates the influence, of (sports) medicine. EiM identifies this as a process of paradigmatic change – 'we must begin to merge the fitness industry with the healthcare industry if we are going to improve the world' – and evokes questions of jurisdictional legitimacy – 'I believe that sports medicine physicians around the world are the best advocates for Exercise is Medicine' (Sallis 2009: 4). EiM can therefore be read as an explicit attempt on the part of (sports) medicine to colonize a sphere of social life that was previously beyond its domain.

Paradoxically, however, EiM extends/refracts surveillance back on to the medical profession, not only encouraging 'physicians and other healthcare providers to be physically active themselves' (Jonas and Phillips 2009: ix), but presenting this as a moral obligation: 'we heartily recommend that, if you are not presently a regular exerciser yourself, you seriously consider becoming one, both for your own benefit and that of your patients' (Jonas 2009: 7). Illustrative of the interconnection between the US and UK PAHP movements, the CEO of NHS England, Simon Stevens, has recently suggested that NHS staff should themselves join gyms, partly in the belief that this would reduce work absenteeism due to ill health, but partly also in the belief that NHS staff should set a 'good example' to their patients (Helm 2014). He himself is reported to have lost 20 kg prior to his move to this post from Vice President of EiM sponsor, *United Health* (Johnson 2016).

Conclusion

PAHP is an exemplar of medicalization at the conceptual level whereby a previously considered natural aspect of the life-course becomes (re-)defined as having inherently medical properties. It is facilitated by a social concern (obesity) that has become classified as a disease, ideologies of the role of the state (neoliberalism) and its convergence with commercial interests. Moreover, it is aligned with contemporary developments in medicine (e.g. fears about the dangers of biomedical interventions, the increasing identification of pre-disease states and the shifting emphasis from cure to management to self-management) and feeds off and into incipient conceptualizations in health. But PAHP also provides opportunities for sports medicine to attain state mandate and licence and enable the professional projects of those who seek to consolidate and expand the role of the specialism. Significant in this regard is the eschewal of medicalization based on the fraught and contested terrain of deviance (SRI) in favour of what have proved to be 'softer' targets. The ubiquity and social valence of PAHP are underpinned by a widespread commitment to the fundamentally problematic sport–health ideology.

But a holistic assessment of medicalization must consider its multi-level impact. Specifically, as we saw in Chapter 2, contemporary challenges to medical dominance include a declining deference towards medicine (and indeed professions in general), heightened concerns about the efficacy of modern biomedicine, and the increasing importance attached to the subjective patient voice and its potential aggregation as lay knowledge. These issues form the basis of Chapters 5 and 6. To begin, we look at the unfulfilled promise of PAHP as we explore the experiences of a cohort who have answered the health imperative by adhering to PAHP, have exercised regularly, but who have become injured as a consequence. How does a medicalization process premised on the disregard of SRI impact on the public and the broader social influence of sports medicine? Second, we look more closely at the EiM agenda and the experiences and attitudes of those who have been medically directed to increase their activity levels for restorative health purposes. How do they receive PAHP messages and how do they integrate these ideas into social practice? In other words, how does medicalization at the conceptual level of PAHP impact on the institutional and interactional levels of sport, medicine and health?

Chapter 5

Medicalization, injury and the exercising public

As discussed in Chapter 4, the intersection of sport, medicine and health has become increasingly evident in recent years through government attempts to persuade the population to become more physically active. In line with the NPH more broadly, PAHP leads to the transfer of the economic burden from the collective to the individual, reproduces social inequalities while boosting the profitability of commercial organizations, and fosters the development of health-oriented lifestyles, which come to dominate identities and social practice (Lupton 1995). In justifying the broad approach of PAHP, the 'benefits' of participation are emphasized while the potential costs – the physical, economic and social consequences of injury – are underestimated or obscured. These trends represent a fairly explicit and intended manifestation of the medicalization of social life which, while largely operative on the conceptual level, has the potential to penetrate deeply into people's lives and consciousness.

In this and the next chapter, we look at the impact of PAHP in terms of its permeation into people's lives and identities. We look first at exercise as preventative medicine and latterly at exercise as a form of treatment. Initially then, the focus is the social implications of 'healthism' (Crawford 2006) and the sport–health ideology for the sector of the population who adhere to PAHP advice and pursue active or sporting lifestyles. While the previous review of epidemiological literature indicated that the direct and indirect costs of SRI were more significant than PAHP materials have come to portray, the methodological approach underpinning epidemiological evidence tends to both overlook 'hard to reach' populations (and hence the concentration of data on EM and GP visits), and the qualitative, lived experience, of illness and injury. Consequently, drawing on the notion of biographical disruption – a 'core' theoretical concept in the sociology of health and illness (Bury 1982; Williams 2000) – this chapter suggests that contrary to their medical representation as minor events, SRI can have a devastating, life-altering, impact indicative of more extreme examples of the social crisis that has been charted in relation to chronic illness. As we will see, in part this is a consequence of the biographical contingencies of sports injury 'patients' including, amongst other things, their conscription to contemporary notions of healthism embracing personal responsibility towards bodily self-management. But it is also partly attributable to the relatively restricted medicalization of sport and exercise which leads those with SRI to largely remain outside the domain of the (sports) medicine profession. Specifically, the consequences of a professional project pursued through a medicalization of life-course events rather than medicalization of deviance (injury) are that this population are forced to pursue alternative and lay-guided treatments for their SRIs.

Biographical disruption

The criteria frequently adopted in epidemiological research – e.g. quantifying direct and indirect costs – illustrate only part of the broader impact of illness or injury. Alternatively, the notion of biographical disruption is premised on the idea that, while illness/disease might be defined as biophysical events which medical professionals seek to 'cure', the 'patient's' subjective experience is much more expansive and can relate more to how the individual and his/her network of relations perceive, respond and live with symptoms of said illness/disease or, in this case, injury. Such qualitative measures provide a better assessment of how severely SRI is experienced; what it really *means* to people.

The notion of biographical disruption was introduced by Mike Bury (1982) in the context of research exploring patients' experiences of arthritis. Bury argued that becoming ill was for many a *critical situation*, which led to three elements of biographical disruption. First, illness disrupts taken-for-granted assumptions and behaviours. Specifically, whereas most of the time we are oblivious to the functioning of our body (it is an 'absent presence'), illness brings our bodily state to the forefront of consciousness. Our malfunctioning bodies are, in this sense, 'dys-eased' (Leder 1990). Second, illness disrupts our explanatory frameworks, leading us to re-think our biography; why me? why now? what has caused this? It leads to a questioning of the sense of self and of one's future trajectory. Third, illness disrupts the way we deploy our resources; physically in terms of our time and effort, financially, and socially in terms of the activities in which we engage. Bury inferred from this that chronic illness had meaning in terms of both practical consequences – for individuals and families there is a cost of giving time and money to manage the illness which impinges on work and home life – and symbolic significance, or the 'profound effect on how individuals regard themselves, and how they think others see them' (Williams 2000: 44).

Bury's work has spawned a myriad of studies which, while frequently stressing the need for a wider-ranging or more nuanced application, build upon rather than reject the basic premise of biographical disruption. For instance, biographical continuity or flow refers to the way illness may be experienced not as 'an imminent invader of everyday life, but rather part of an ongoing life story' (Faircloth *et al.* 2004: 244), while biographical reinforcement refers to the way in which chronic illness can make a pre-existing identity even stronger (Carricaburu and Pierret 1995). A more intense level of distress has been described as biographical abruption, or disruption so severe that it entails a sudden ending or a breaking off from normal life by people simply unable to imagine how life can go on (Locock *et al.* 2009). Finally, biographical repair or reinstatement refers to the incorporation of illness into 'normal' life, for instance by embracing the impairment, (re-)defining life as normal, minimizing the social consequences of illness, or engaging in behaviour designed to demonstrate normalcy to others (Sanderson *et al.* 2011). While the notion of disruption is 'intrinsically negative' (Locock *et al.* 2009: 1045), there is 'an implicit moral acceptance of normalisation as good' (Sanderson *et al.* 2011: 620).

All studies, however, accept the idea that social context is a particularly significant mediator of the impact of biomedical diagnosis (Bury 2001). Monaghan and Gabe (2015: 3) argue that '[W]hether a chronic illness is suffered … on any occasion depends on multiple context-dependent [biographical] contingencies' such as age, class, gender, social deprivation and co-morbidities. However, in one of the more prominent critiques of biographical disruption, Williams (2000) calls for more work on the relationship between illness, biographical disruption and social reflexivity, citing health promotion, screening and surveillance as responsible for invoking a kind of 'body McCarthyism' in 'late modernity' as citizens are 'increasingly advised and instructed, encouraged and cajoled, on how best to manage ourselves and ride the emotional waves of everyday life' (Williams 2000: 57). Thus, we need to ask to what extent does SRI entail biographical disruption, to what extent does this relate to NPH and PAHP, and what are the implications of this for the medicalization of sport? In order to answer these questions data from a series of interviews conducted with participants in sport and exercise who had experience of SRI will be explored (see Appendix).

Attitudes towards sport-related injury

At the outset, it should be noted that those who took part in this research exhibited a predictably middle-class bias. Most of the respondents possessed or were studying for higher education qualifications while many had occupations either in the educational sector or described as 'managerial'. A shop assistant, receptionist, HGV driver and motor mechanic represented lower socio-economic occupations. This bias was predictable in that the link between physical activity and social class is well-documented (Eime *et al.* 2015), but it further illustrates that PAHP is typical of health promotional campaigns more generally, which are most effective in reaching socially and economically privileged groups and thus frequently perpetuate the social inequalities that both structure and include health (Baum and Fisher 2014).

Moreover, due to the sampling techniques employed, most interviewees closely aligned with specific sports. These included the contact sports that epidemiological surveys indicate have the highest prevalence of injury (e.g. martial arts, rugby union), non-contact team and individual sports in which injury has been shown to be less frequent (e.g. volleyball, athletics/ running) and newer and lifestyle sports (e.g. roller derby, kitesurfing). Three respondents described engagement in a range of sport-related activities, indicative of a physically active or 'sporting' identity contoured by the inherent logic of PAHP. While the conflation of sport, exercise and physical activity is of course a problematic aspect of both the policy environment and sport–health ideology more generally, our emphasis here is on the qualitative depth of the SRI experience. While SRI may be more common in relation to certain groups of activity, it is not exclusive to any single type.

While the research aimed to explore everyday minor ailments as much as the more severe injuries, inevitably there was a further bias towards the latter in interviewees' accounts. The majority of injuries described were musculoskeletal, affecting joints (elbow, knee, shoulder), ligaments, tendons, cartilage and muscles. Interviewees either spoke of definitively diagnosed – broken vertebrae, broken pelvis, anterior cruciate ligament injuries, dislocation of the posterior tibial tendon, etc. – or more loosely defined conditions – overuse shoulder injury, hamstring injury, knee injury, ongoing neural pain. This reflected both an individuals' degree of physiological interest and understanding but also their history, perception and recollection of medical encounters.

The frequency of injury did broadly correlate with the types of sport/ exercise undertaken and thus partly mirrored epidemiological findings. For instance, martial artists noted that making coaches and other fighters aware of one's injuries was a routine part of training. A participant described using a herbal treatment to reduce bruising 'all the time', or needing ibuprofen on a regular, perhaps weekly, basis. Similarly, a rugby player stated that there was 'not a ... player that's not carrying an injury', and described the need to consume 'quite a lot of painkillers just to get yourself through'. When asked about the medical demands associated with the sport, it was estimated that, in 12 years, 'I reckon I've been to A&E [Emergency Medicine] 30 times with either myself or with a friend; easily 30, probably 40 actually'. This equates to 2.5–3.25 times per year.

Those who took part in the kind of non-contact sports that epidemiological research suggests have a lower injury incidence, described the management of chronic injury as routine. This was either contextualized in relation to an individual's commitment to the sport – 'when you train so much you've got to kind of accept that at some point something's going to go wrong' (volleyball player) – or more frequently the ageing process. Thus, a netballer reflected on the constant 'fire-fighting' of 'niggles';

> I wish I was 19 again … I'm quite realistic that if I didn't want to have niggles, I'd have to be training full time and not working and that's just not feasible … So it's kind of something that you just have to accept as part of the course.

Similarly, an interviewee who participated in a range of sports/physical activities reflected,

> as you get older you get used to having niggles all the time (laughs) … I guess mainly just the odd tweak in the calf, or may be just general aching after doing something I've not done for a while.

These comments reflect a pattern with musculoskeletal disorders whereby, 'pain frequently emerges amidst the activities of daily living and pain management becomes routinised' (Morden *et al.* 2015: 894).

But perhaps the central characteristic of the SRI experiences of the exercising public was its ongoing and/or escalating nature. A cricketer described how a calf muscle injury led to deep vein thrombosis and blood clots on the lung, a runner described how after seven months a suspected sprained ankle was diagnosed as a detached ankle tendon, and a third interviewee described how two years of Achilles tendonitis resulted in lower back pain, sacroiliac or SI joint pain (a joint in the pelvis) and a hamstring injury. The most extensive list of injuries was provided by an interviewee who, over the years, had taken part in a variety of sports ranging from rounders to triathlon to kitesurfing to judo. This interviewee described multiple injuries: 'loose ankles' (ligament instability that can lead to frequent sprains); prolotherapy to her back, neck and pubic area (injections to stimulate the tendons or ligaments to relieve pain); hip 'problems'; groin surgery; and surgical removal of part of the shoulder joint. The developmental pattern of SRIs makes them particularly difficult to epidemiologically chart because they are not conducive to the identification of a specific aetiology.

An inherent element of this, and indeed one of the most universally cited themes, was the expression of attitudes towards injury which replicated what has previously been described as the 'culture of risk' (e.g. Frey 1991; see Chapter 1). For example, interviewees talked about carrying on when feeling injured but not necessarily in pain (including concussed), or about continuing despite what they described as intense pain. A cricketer relayed the occurrence of what turned out to be an Achilles injury in the following way: 'I've never felt any pain like that before … [I thought] "I've done something really bad here, but I'll carry on"'. Those taking part in more institutionalized forms of sport discussed the extrinsic pressures to play through pain and with injury. For instance some talked about being persuaded by their coach to carry on training even though they knew they had an injury, while a martial artist who injured knee cartilage during training described how they carried on training for 'a few months,... [but] had to adapt how I was training. I was competing so I had to continue'. Typically, a runner stated that 'I think I'd always try to wait until the end of the season' before attempting to rest or resolve a SRI.

Such behaviour was widely depicted as normal for those active in sport. Thus, in recalling a failure to respond to warning signs of pain a runner said, 'as usual, that's what I normally do if I feel pain or aching, and you just don't think about it much, "just keep going", and I did'. Similarly, another said, 'I can remember there were sessions where I was running and I was kind of wincing as I'm taking steps and thinking "well, I really shouldn't be doing this", but you kind of go with it'. Such attitudes were not just confined to those more deeply immersed in the sports culture of risk. As one interviewee who had taken up jogging 3 months earlier having not exercised for about 10 years, said; 'I did the normal thing where you rest it for a bit, and it feels better again so you start running on it again and it hurts again'. Drawing an explicit contrast between those who take part in sport and those who don't, a rugby player argued that, 'the boundaries that athletes have for pain and the discomfort and damage that they're willing to do to their body, is different to what a normal person would be willing to accept'.

A central reason why this behaviour was both widespread and normalized lies in the degree to which there are elements of convergence between the philosophies of the culture of risk and the NPH. For example, interviewees did unthinkingly continue to exercise while in pain due to an internalization of both the social desirability of keeping active and the sport–health ideology, manifest here in the lack of concern that continued participation could lead to (more) serious impairment. For instance, one interviewee reflected that they should perhaps not have been 'quite so enthusiastic' in undertaking rehabilitative exercises, while a volleyball player explained their behaviour thus:

> The mentality? Why not? Why not keep going if you can? If you can move. And I guess you just keep going anyway. Because I thought I'm too busy to do proper physio and I want to keep playing and I can move. I can still jump. I can still do these things. I'll just do it.

But others exhibited various aspects of an identity characteristically formed under 'healthism' and the PAHP mediation of NPH in particular. For instance, an interviewee who became injured in the process of completing a first marathon combined an internalization of a 'more is better' philosophy with a mixture of euphoria and social distinction from participating in this 'most visible contemporary spectacle of health' (Nettleton and Hardey 2006: 457). Consequently, this led him to 'keep going ... whack some painkillers down' and worsen the injury. The elusiveness, yet social reward, of attaining 'fitness' led others to defy recommendations to rest their injured body. A runner explained,

> I'll be honest with you, I couldn't face ... just mentally the thought of easing off for 2 or 3 months was a bit much ... and whether I'd made things a bit worse by trying to run after 4 weeks, I don't know.

Others exhibited the force of a quest for exciting significance, expressing the desire to create meaning through sports participation ('[I] just kept trying to salvage it [the season]'), or pursuing happiness even if this was at the expense of health (attempting to run, surf and snowboard, while ignoring an injury that would subsequently require surgery). A fourth group reflected the stigmatization associated with non-compliance to NPH as SRI served to undermine personal self-worth in a range of ways. Interviewees expressed guilt in relation to: having ignored the early signs of injury and consequently exacerbating the condition; taking time off work for an injury that was seen as 'avoidable'; 'failing' to attend to the usual demands of a young family while being 'sat around for a couple of days ... [when I] didn't actually feel ill'; and turning into 'a bit of a slob' and entering a spiral of inactivity and weight gain. Some even explicitly used the language of neoliberal ideologies of productivity to explain their behaviour: 'I think that's the reason why I keep trying to play – to try and you know, still use time productively'.

Thus, this cohort experienced frequent SRI. Often, subsequent behaviours aggravated existing 'niggles' or led to additional or alternative impediments. There is some evidence to suggest that such mentality is a derivative of the culture of risk seen in elite and competitive sport more broadly, but again interviewees spoke in terms that revealed the aspects of population surveillance which critics have identified as part of the NPH, and the specific problems of PAHP derived from the imprecise and elusive goals of 'fitness' as health. Tellingly, people's exercise patterns bore little relationship to the kind of moderate, rhythmic and gentle exercise patterns most conducive to health gains and sought, instead, more meaningful sporting experiences that were defined as socially and emotionally gratifying; more vigorous, longer duration or believed to facilitate thinness. These accounts very much run counter to the claims that taking part in exercise entails a 'very low risk of injury' (AMRC 2015) and that such risks 'tend to be overestimated' (RCP 2012: 6), but in the next section we look to explore the relative severity of SRI experiences.

Biographical disruption and sport-related injury

Some of the injuries that interviewees reported could be said, relative to biomedical criteria, to be particularly severe. For instance, a rugby player reported breaking two vertebrae after being hit by an opponent during a fight and subsequently could not work for 14 weeks. Similarly, an accident in which a kitesurfer was blown into a harbour wall resulted in a broken pelvis (in three places), broken ribs, a ripped bowel, a prolapsed disc, a dislocated knee, surgical reconstruction of an anterior cruciate ligament, a neck injury and nerve damage. But across the sample it was also evident that interviewees experienced multiple facets of biographical disruption – altered experiences, resources, outlook – many of which illustrated that SRI could have deep and significant ramifications.

The extent to which SRI disrupted the individual's taken-for-granted assumptions and behaviours was evident both in the phenomenological experience of injury, and its holistic impact on daily lives. The pain many interviewees associated with SRI disrupted the body's 'absent presence' (Leder 1990) and ranged from 'excruciating, to the point where I'm still actually bracing myself when I go upstairs', to more of a 'continuous aggravation ... you kind of get used to it hurting all the time'. Moreover, the impact of sports injury was frequently omnipresent: 'all the time I'm conscious of it. I know that I've been sat here for kind of two, three minutes, and I can already feel that I should probably be moving the position that I'm in because it starts to get uncomfortable'. The effect of pain 'wears you down, it does make you quite tired, and sometimes you're at the point where you just think I wish this pain would go away'. Pain relief was therefore ubiquitous, either to manage sports participation or facilitate sleep. Typically, interviewees conveyed the sense that the disruption associated with pain and pain management 'takes over your life', as 'it becomes part of you and you probably don't realise what pain you're in until it goes away'.

This led previously habitual behaviour to become fundamentally problematized. For this reason the disruption that SRI could cause to an exerciser's self-identity might best be described as biographical abruption, for many imagined 'life simply not happening at all – the story is already over' (Locock et al. 2009: 1048). For instance, one volleyball player described how injury meant that their life had changed from being centred on four training/playing sessions a week to 'nothing, absolutely nothing'. For many, training had created a 'very routine life' and thus injury necessarily entailed 'disruption to your whole routine'. Injury could deprive exercisers of the primary source of pleasure in their lives:

> I had something in a way to look forward to, every day. I'd turn up at the track, probably been crying all the way here, and then I'd run and

I was in a different world ... the injury really affected me ... I just lost everything – I lost the routine and didn't really know what to do with myself.

(Runner)

Another stated that 'Everything I enjoy doing I just couldn't do'. The identity-defining character of sports participation was encapsulated by one interviewee who recalled his gym attendance prior to injury: 'It wasn't just a sport, it was like a lifestyle because obviously, you change the way you eat and whatever' and, due to body modification, 'there was a bit of an ego issue as well'.

SRI also entailed a considerable disruption to the injured exerciser's mobilization of resources. This could be financial (some interviewees had either ceased or changed employment; the use of private healthcare is discussed further below), temporal (albeit generating a surfeit rather than a scarcity of time) but, most importantly, in terms of social dislocation manifest in a sense of lost freedom and loneliness. Interviewees contrasted their injury state to the liberating phenomenological experience of sports participation (Hockey and Allen-Collinson 2009). A runner described how an injury would fundamentally disrupt their planned holiday:

> [it's] just heart-breaking to be honest. I mean where we stay is in the middle of a forest. It's absolutely beautiful because it literally is in the middle of a forest. It's just lovely, and to not be able to run, [pause] I waited and waited and I thought 'I'll give it a go,' [because] I was so down in the mouth.

But physical impairment was also often accompanied by strained social relations. Interviewees described how their partners or family members 'hate it' when they are injured, and find them difficult to live with. An interviewee whose partner (also) frequently exercised observed that injury threatened the shared interest which was central to their relationship. A former gym user reflected on the constraints experienced through a loss of confidence;

> when you see your body changing and getting smaller and fatter ... I don't like taking my top off now. And also like [when I] socialise as well, with girls and stuff. I don't feel confident going up to someone and talking to them.

The social dislocation that stemmed from changes to the use of leisure time was further evident in the antagonism the injured expressed towards their friends. As one recalled, '[I was] having arguments with everyone around me'. Indeed, the injured actually found little solace in the attempts of those around them to acknowledge their 'illness' and thus legitimate their 'sick role' (Parsons 1975):

> That's one of the most annoying things that someone that is not injured can try to do ... [They would] say, 'Oh I understand what you're going through'. I was thinking, 'No you don't', because you know, there you are playing, you're jumping ... [it] feeds that kind of envy.
>
> (Netballer)

Another interviewee described the contradictory emotional consequences of trying to maintain a normal routine by doing rehabilitation exercises at their usual volleyball training session:

> Everyone was amazing. All the girls were super supportive ... [but] whilst I was doing my little exercises and they were playing volleyball just next to me ... I had thoughts such as, 'I hate you all and you don't know how lucky you are because you can jump, and you can run, and you can move'.

Managing sports injury, therefore, can be 'burdensome, necessitating "hard and heavy work" including physical, relational and social capital' (Moore *et al.* 2015: 4).

Finally, disruption to explanatory frameworks was evident in the fears interviewees expressed about how a current SRI could permanently shape their future. A volleyball player stated that 'I just think I'll be limited ... [the injury] makes me accept that I'll be limited forever'. A cricketer argued that

> At the moment I can't see a point in the future where I'm going to be 100% fit. I think I'm always going to carry an injury at least like somewhere in my legs ... I just don't see any light at the end of the tunnel.

The incidence of SRI was seen to be 'unfair' and only resolution of a current injury would 'let me get my life back'. Sports injury could therefore lead to a fundamental re-structuring of both one's sense of self and future trajectory. A runner justified the financial burden of sourcing private healthcare in terms of 'maintaining me as a person'. A number of interviewees explicitly reflected 'why me?'

From the above we can see that, in addition to the ongoing and frequent experience of SRI, exercisers experience a range of biographically disrupting patterns, some of which depict SRI as a particularly critical situation within an individual's life. While attempts to precisely quantify the relative financial and social costs of illness and injury may be fundamentally questionable, there is nothing in this qualitative account that would contradict estimates that the latter constitutes 81% or more of total SRI costs (Finch *et al.* 2001; Weaver *et al.* 1999). However, inherent to the amelioration of biographical disruption and thus severity of illness/injury is biographical repair, the aspect of SRI that we turn to next.

Sport-related injury and biographical repair

In order to resolve biographical disruption/abruption it is necessary for the ill or injured to undergo aspects of biographical, if not physical, repair. Fundamentally, the notion of biographical repair revolves around the notion of normalcy (Sanderson *et al.* 2011). However, in the context of SRI, biographical repair has particular characteristics, for these conditions are (generally) not life-threatening and (certainly longer-term) do not preclude people from the 'normal' (i.e. relatively physically inactive) lives of the majority of western populations. However, the interviewees did not speak of creating normalcy as participants in other studies of biographical disruption have (e.g. compensatory attempts to seek pleasure in other aspects of life (Locock *et al.* 2009), adjusting their lifestyle/pace to incorporate their condition (Sanderson *et al.* 2011)) for what constitutes 'normal' for exercisers centres upon their return to sport/exercise participation. In their attempts to attain this, the injured are hindered by broader social discourses of the importance of exercise and the body, a sense of failed or compromised ability to self-manage health and, especially, the limited (and/or ineffectual) healthcare support available to them which stems from a limited medicalization of this aspect of sport.

Given the degree of biographical disruption identified above, interviewees clearly had strong motives for seeking treatment. Where injured exercisers found that simply carrying on, taking painkillers, etc., was unsatisfactory they became proactive in prognosis- if not treatment-shopping, trying to persuade healthcare professionals to sanction their intentions to resume sports participation, phoning their GP to see if they could/should start to train again, or getting cortisol injections as a 'short-term fix' to enable them to 'continue to play'. But, overall, few pursued this strategy and only did so when their injuries were particularly severe. Rather, a range of reasons were provided to explain why those with SRIs were dissuaded from seeking medical help. Like musculoskeletal injuries more generally, many were self-treated as interviewees' general experiences were that healthcare professionals found such disorders 'difficult to diagnose precisely and treat effectively' (Bushby *et al.* 1997: 84). However, a perceived lack of medical expertise, and a sense that GPs were 'just not interested', compounded these trends. For instance a runner recalled her experience of primary and secondary care as 'totally unhelpful' in treating her daughter's sports injury, while another intimated that scepticism was embedded in the lay knowledge of sport communities, explaining that they had not sought medical treatment because, 'I just thought they'll just say rest or something, from what people told me like'. Rugby players similarly reported a lack of effective medical resolution as GPs would typically say 'it's just bruised', or 'Just take painkillers. If it keeps getting worse come back and see me'. In particular, concern was expressed in relation to the speed with which interviewees thought GPs would seek to timetable their recovery. An interviewee recalled deciding not to consult a GP but to 'carry on' until a competition was complete, while another described the recommendation to take 12 weeks off from sport as 'just not practical'. The sample therefore reflected Baarveld *et al.*'s (2011: 32) synopsis; 'patients with a sports-related injury that consult a GP are mostly diagnosed non-specifically and receive mainly explanation and medical advice for their injury'. This aspect of the exercisers' world was, therefore, fundamentally *un*-medicalized.

Interviewees believed that medicine could not help them partly because the medical system was primarily orientated to get people back to work (rather than living their lives 'normally') and partly because physicians viewed injured exercisers as partly culpable for their own predicament. For example, one person stated that they're 'not going to prioritise me because I'm an athlete', while another described a very unsatisfactory experience of being seen by an MSK specialist:

> I went and saw this person and ... she was just like 'oh, right, so you've been running?'
> 'Yeah I've been running.'
> 'Alright, OK, so what's the problem?'
> I was like 'the problem's not that I can't run.' ... and I was like I knew this would happen ... she didn't quite get it.... She almost laughed at me, like, 'But you're active, What's the problem?'

Alongside this indifference to, or incomprehension of, the 'problems' of those with SRI was a perception of judgemental attitudes towards what might be perceived to contain elements of 'self-harm'. A martial artist recalled that GPs were 'sometimes disapproving', while another interview said that the attitude towards rugby players in EM departments was 'like "oh no, not again"'. A third argued that if you attend EM with a sports injury 'they put you at the back of the queue'. Medical personnel were therefore perceived to range from uninterested in expanding their jurisdictional realm to resistant to requests to legitimize the 'deviance' of SRI.

Three options were available to injured exercisers who viewed the available medical treatment as unsatisfactory. The first, self-treatment, could be based on knowledge acquired through health-related qualifications, or 'simply having been all my life surrounded by athletes and players and in uni. and school and so I've known a lot of people who have done it before and described it [the injury], how I felt'. However, it was clear that self-treatment was often fuelled by frustration at the suspension in a non-normal life. Monthly appointments with an NHS physiotherapist were found to be, 'just too long to be left on your own ... I start wandering off and looking at the internet and trying to find solutions myself [laughs] ... I've diagnosed myself with all sorts of things [laughs]'. Second, the injured frequently acquired help from family, friends and fellow athletes. One interviewee described how a teammate who was also a physiotherapist,

> suggested that if it was a torn muscle, then they wouldn't do anything for me in the hospital ... 'they're going to give you a pain killer and they're going to say you've got to not put any weight on that leg for three days. You're going to wait in hospital. You're going to be in pain'.

Others argued that the relative merits of lay and medical knowledge were not clear: 'people that have been in martial arts for 20 years might know more about the injuries than a doctor possibly'. A second martial artist had themselves become recognized as a mini-expert on injuries within their sport; 'They all come to me actually. I've got sort of sprays, creams, you name it, I've got it in my bag'. Finally, injured exercisers had the option of paying for private medical care. Indeed, 16 of the 20 interviewees had, at some point, paid for treatments ranging from one-off surgical procedures, to ongoing care from physiotherapists, psychologists, massage and sports therapists and a range of CAM providers such as osteopaths, chiropractors, and acupuncture. The main motives for seeking private medical help reflected the extant literature (Knill-Jones 1997) and included the timing of treatment to enable people to work or practice their sport unhindered, and perceptions that sports specialist healthcare providers had greater expertise and more 'sympathy and empathy' for/with the injured athlete. Interviewees especially liked healthcare providers who asked them about the particular movements required in their sport, emphasized the importance of remaining active in a way that they saw as constructive (for their future sport participation), or explicitly oriented treatment towards a point at which the patient would return to play (RTP).

Thus, the behaviours of this cohort were indicative of a challenge to medical dominance. The injured exerciser relies on a relatively coherent and organized body of lay knowledge (which itself appropriates aspects of medical knowledge) and engages with a range of 'alternative' medical providers (both in the sense of CAMS and outside of mainstream provision) due to a disenchantment with the efficacy of (aspects of) biomedicine. Fundamentally, though, these patients do not want this degree of control over their own health/illness (Lupton 1997). While often driven by feelings of desperation – 'if there was anything at all that would have helped I'd have done it' – engagement with these medical providers was favourably viewed not simply because it was seen to alleviate the patient's physical problems, but because they aligned with the ideologies of PAHP and the broader health imperative to remain active.

Conclusion

From the above, we can see that even if sports injuries generally have relatively limited biophysical consequences (a view problematized by the epidemiological findings), regular exercisers experience SRI as frequent and significant in social and biographical terms. This may be indicative of the growing social intolerance of minor ailments that has helped drive medicalization (Conrad 2007), but the degree of disruption/abruption stemming from these non-terminal and relatively minor 'life-limiting' conditions also partly relates to the context and circumstance in which these conditions are subjectively experienced. Largely middle class, relatively youthful (if not necessarily young) and with self-perceptions of general good health and desirable body shapes, this group had high life expectations and relatively little experience of coping with diversity (Williams 2000). But, perhaps most significantly, they had previously enjoyed a degree of social distinction through their participation in leisure activities, which accrued a reflected virtue. The primary (social) consequence of SRI was to remove the individual not only from an activity that they personally enjoyed, but from an activity that was valued as a consequence of its broader social valence through embodied health status and reflected moral worth. These individuals went from exemplars to conspicuous failures of health self-management; from strongly conforming, to feeling unable to undertake responsible citizenship; from having 'correct' choices embedded into lifestyle to finding such choices were evidently unobtainable. If, as the *Exercise is Medicine* advocates suggest, being active 'makes you feel better', 'makes you look better'; and 'makes you feel better about yourself' (Jonas 2009: 5), the enforced inactivity as a consequence of SRI makes you feel worse, look worse and feel worse about yourself.

The difficulties this community encounter stem from the intersection of two processes. The interdependent relations and knowledge production process behind PAHP lead one fundamental but unintended outcome to be overlooked; given the epidemiology of SRI and the continued conflation of sport, exercise and physical activity, a direct consequence of the success of PAHP will be an increase not only in health costs but also the number of people unable to exercise and therefore adhere to health advice. Evidence is emerging to suggest that this is a tangible problem. For instance, according to *Sport England* data, 'injury' is the fifth most frequently cited reason (17%) why people no longer participate in sport (Sport England

2012). Moreover 42% of those who had ceased sports participation due to SRI stated that they were 'not at all' or 'not very' likely to participate in their sport again. Similarly, an Australian study found that, 'serious sport and active recreation injuries have large, negative, persistent impacts on participants' physical activity levels, independent of functional recovery' (Andrew *et al*. 2014: 377). A year after incurring a sports injury, just 40 to 65% of patients had returned to sports participation and, of those who had not, relatively few 'compensated' by replacing sport with less vigorous activities (e.g. walking). Return to sports participation was particularly poor amongst lower socio-economic groups. But an additional problem is the partial or incomplete medicalization of sport, for medicalization at the conceptual level in terms of PAHP is not matched by medicalization at the institutional or interactional levels. The role of the unintended consequences of PAHP – a form of public health with a potentially unique self-defeating logic – not only means that the compliant are statistically likely to require additional medical support, but that the subsequent failure to self-manage health further fuels biographical disruption. PAHP not only creates citizens who self-manage their health, but also who have to self-manage the *ill*-health that stems from their attempts to self-manage due to the lack of more comprehensive medicalization. We look at the barriers to such self-management in Chapter 6.

Chapter 6

Is exercise medicine?

The lived experience of physical activity in healthcare

Chapter 4 briefly introduced the EiM movement, the explicit aim of which is, 'To make physical activity and exercise a standard part of a disease prevention and treatment medical paradigm in the United States' (Jonas and Philips 2009: ix). The rationale for EiM is that exercise (sufficient to induce slight breathlessness, enabling one to talk but not sing) is 'the much needed vaccine to prevent chronic disease and premature death' (Sallis 2009: 3). Moreover, the 'exercise pill' is claimed to have miraculous effects; 'If we had a pill that conferred all the confirmed health benefits of exercise would we not do everything humanly possible to see to it that everyone had access to this wonder drug?' (Sallis 2009: 3). While it is conceded that 'either too much or too little [exercise] can be harmful' (Phillips *et al.* 2009a 149) EiM replicates ideas that 'the more intense the activity, that is the more aerobic it is, the more benefit there is to be gained from it' (Jonas 2009: 11). For this reason clinicians are exhorted to 'collectively urge *all* patients to become *more* active and stay active throughout their lives' (Sallis 2009: 4, emphasis added). EiM has been so influential that it is now established in 43 countries, and its inaugural 'World Congress' (2010) was attended by delegates from over 60 countries (Neville 2013).

EiM embodies the psychologization of PAHP (Horrocks and Johnson 2014) and lifestyle drift (Popay *et al.* 2010), focusing on 'change and how to make it, choices to be made and how to make them' (Jonas 2009: 1). There are expressed desires to create a 'broad awareness' of the desirability of exercise (Jonas and Philips 2009: ix), but also an attempt to provide clinicians with the tools and techniques to effectively make these changes. A central aspect of this educational work has been the publication of a book which, in many ways, is an instruction manual for those charged with implementing EiM, the *ACSM's Exercise is Medicine: A Clinician's Guide to Exercise Prescription* (Jonas and Philips 2009). Containing guidance for advising/persuading patients of the benefits of regular physical activity, it draws only briefly on the clinical evidence for the reduction of risk and/or effective management of certain conditions and emphasizes in particular aesthetic and lifestyle factors related to exercise including the claim that

'Regular exercise can be fun, if you let it be fun!' (Jonas 2009: 5–6). Similarly, included amongst the seven major benefits of taking regular exercise, is the advice that it 'can help you feel younger and act that way too' and 'can help spark your sex life'; exercise 'is the only way to "get in shape"' (Jonas 2009: 6). The (in)decision to be physically (in)active is projected as an essentially personal and individual (ir)responsibility. Clinicians are advised that their 'patient ... knows that he "should" be more active' (Phillips *et al.* 2009b: 91).

Previously, we saw the multiple senses in which EiM represents a form of medicalization: effectively redefining an everyday social practice under a medical rubric; explicitly expanding and consolidating the jurisdictional influence of medicine over both citizens and the fitness industry; and even refracting medical surveillance back onto the profession itself. As these factors largely operate at the conceptual level, it is necessary to ask what broader impact such policies have on people's lives. Thus, in this chapter, we seek to explore the literal claim of EiM, and a claim that is implicit in PAHP more generally, that undertaking exercise medicinally contributes to the relief of human suffering (Edwards and McNamee 2006). Specifically, how does the reality of exercise experienced at the interactional level relate to these claims for EiM?

The empirical focus of this chapter is the lived experience of health/ illness of a group of 26 people who have been diagnosed with Chronic Obstructive Pulmonary Disease (COPD) (see Appendix). COPD patient's experiences of, and attitudes toward, physical activity provide an excellent case study of the broader EiM and NPH movements for three reasons. First, given the centrality of exercise to COPD treatment programmes, this cohort had either been explicitly advised or were acutely conscious of the (clinical) desirability of exercise. Second, given the demographic profile of COPD sufferers this cohort illustrates some of the more extreme physical (and to some extent social) disadvantages and thus tests the extent to which *all* patients can become more active. Third, the role of smoking in the aetiology of COPD centrally locates the illness in lifestyle-centred explanations of health and thus magnifies the potential dual role of self-responsibility and guilt in the contemporary illness experience. In other words this cohort will both directly medically benefit from exercise and be acutely aware of the health imperative (Lupton 1995).

As we will see, while those diagnosed with COPD had largely internalized broader cultural messages that stem from PAHP's medicalization of sport and exercise, the impact of these conceptual developments was significantly constrained by the problems encountered when trying to implement such messages at the interactional level of behavioural change. The chapter illustrates how PAHP depictions of the choice(s) to exercise are simply unrealistic and fundamentally at odds with the physical and structural barriers individuals face. It therefore concludes that EiM, and PAHP more generally, is indicative of an imperialistic form of medicalization which, to some extent, creates iatrogenesis as it exacerbates the everyday lived experiences of those diagnosed with COPD.

Chronic obstructive pulmonary disease, illness narratives and physical activity

COPD entails airflow obstruction, which gets progressively worse and cannot be fully reversed or 'cured'. Smoking tobacco is believed to be the main cause of COPD with approximately 90% of COPD patients having smoked during their lives. Consequently, COPD disproportionately affects males from lower socio-economic groups (Hansen *et al.* 2007). The patient experience of COPD is complicated by the fact that onset rarely coincides with either subjective perception or presentation of physical symptoms. When manifest, primary physical symptoms include chronic coughing and sputum production (V. Williams *et al.* 2011). At less severe levels of the illness the lack of oxygen intake can lead to feelings of lethargy/tiredness, confusion, forgetfulness and irritability. While COPD patients frequently negotiate the 'oxygen cost' of particular activities (Lindqvist and Hallberg 2010), they tend also to reject the label of illness or disability, attributing their physical condition to getting old or being out of shape. Indeed, as the symptoms are more-or-less common (associated with a common cold or rationalized in lay epidemiological terms as a 'smokers cough') those with the illness are frequently faced with the dilemma of whether to disclose their diagnosis to others. At more severe levels, patients can experience a sense of social isolation or stagnation (of the physical, social or self), dyspnea (an elemental fear of breathlessness akin to suffocation (Bailey 2004)) and potentially depression. Paradoxically, the symptoms of COPD create a cycle of reduced physical activity. It is predicted that by 2030 COPD will be the fourth leading cause of mortality, morbidity and disability worldwide (Boeckxstaens *et al.* 2012).

While traditionally treatment for COPD has focused on smoking cessation and inhaler medication, increasing emphasis is being placed on pulmonary rehabilitation (PR) and exercise. It is widely (clinically) recognized that COPD patients can accrue a range of health benefits from taking part in PR, including reduced breathlessness, improved muscle strength, and improved management of exacerbations leading to enhanced quality of life, reduced healthcare costs and extended life expectancy. However both uptake for and completion of PR are poor (Williams 2011). The following have been identified as barriers to physical activity for patients with COPD: personal issues (low prioritization/being busy, health fears or anxiety/depression); changing health status (fluctuating symptoms and co-morbidities); lack of support; ongoing smoking; and external factors (environmental and logistical problems) (Thorpe *et al.* 2012). A weakness with the research in this area is that it generally focuses on PR rather than physical activity and exercise as part of patients' everyday lived experience, indicative of the tendency for such research to favour easily accessible rather than qualitatively meaningful populations.

The typology of biographical disruption discussed in Chapter 5 can be usefully augmented by the concept of illness narratives (Bury 2001). Illness narratives help to illustrate how COPD patients experience and represent their experiences of illness in distinct ways. The central premises of exploring patients' narratives of illness are: (a) that what people tell themselves about the experience of illness is equally or more important than the physiological experience; and (b) that the range of narrative strategies an individual has to draw upon are influenced by our social location and experience (e.g. gender, class, knowledge). Probably the most widely used and well known typology of illness narratives appears in the work of Arthur Frank (1995). While Frank argues that there are many different types of narrative, three are particularly important in relation to contemporary illness: chaos, quest and restitution. If the dominant narrative is that of chaos (see biographical abruption, Chapter 5), a person will portray a sense of being out of control, will struggle to understand what is happening to them, and frequently report unexplained symptoms and clinical and/ or social rejection. In a predominantly quest narrative (biographical reinforcement), illness is interpreted as a challenge to be confronted, an impetus for change or as culminating in a broader purpose. Finally, Frank identifies the restitution narrative. He argues that because there is an expectation that this is the narrative that others will want to hear, it is the dominant illness narrative in Western cultures. The restitution narrative (biographical continuity or flow) is based on the assumption that the body will return to its former state/self, but that it is the duty of the sufferer to resolve illness (Frank 1995). It can be summarized as the belief that 'yesterday I was healthy, today I am sick, but tomorrow I will be healthy again'. The restitution narrative is most common amongst the recently ill who perceive themselves as experiencing a temporary and possibly unlucky state, as opposed to those who may see chronic illness as more-or-less permanent and potentially partially self-inflicted. Notably, however, it was rarely invoked by the cohort discussed in Chapter 5 who had or had experienced injuries through sports/exercise participation.

COPD patients exhibit four primary narratives (challenge, chaos, contrary and coping), which closely correspond to Frank's (1995) tripartite schema. The dominant narratives of the challenge and chaos groups closely relate to Arthur Frank's quest and chaos narratives with the former proactive in confronting the limitations of their illness and the latter portraying a sense of incoherence and lack of control. The contrary and coping groups represent a variant of Frank's restitution narrative that is contoured by the knowledge of the impossibility of recovery. Rather than signalling expectations of getting better, these narratives largely functioned to 'exonerate the individual from blame, and help to maintain self worth' (Bury 2001: 275).

The display of these narrative themes closely relates to perceptions of, and participation in, exercise both as a leisure choice and for medicinal purposes. Physical activity was fundamental to the lifestyles of the challenge group with each interviewee reporting frequent engagement in vigorous exercise including cycling, dancing, playing football, and gardening. All in the chaos group perceived that physical activity would be beneficial to their health, but ultimately none exhibited the capacity to routinely exercise. The contrary group were similarly inactive but viewed physical activity with less importance, while the coping group stressed the continued role of exercise (or activity) in their lives, but in line with a broader philosophy of 'getting by' or 'keeping going'. They prioritized the desirability/necessity of physical activity at their 'own pace' which, therefore, frequently meant that they did not meet the minimum breathlessness threshold to be beneficial to health. The narrative, however, enabled them to represent themselves as complying with the *health imperative*.

It was clearly the case, therefore, that attitudes and actions taken to increase physical activity levels through exercise were fundamentally affected by the broader sense in which illness related to biographical disruption and the illness narrative. However, in the next two sections of this chapter, the aim is to assess the lived experience of PAHP and to do this it is useful to explore this cohort as a whole. A notable characteristic of this patient group, and in striking contrast to those patients discussed in Chapter 5, was their relative deprivation with just three having continued in full-time education after the age of 18, and the majority ($n = 15$) having annual earnings below £31,000. In light of this contextual information, here we seek to ascertain: (a) the extent to which a 'broad awareness' of the desirability of exercise has been engendered through PAHP; and (b) the social constraints experienced when those diagnosed with illness make choices about the use of exercise for medicinal purposes. Interviews with COPD patients clearly show that while many harbour generally positive attitudes towards exercise, thereby signalling their consciousness of the health imperative, the barriers to their successful compliance with PAHP strategies form a 'complex web of concerns' (Prior et al. 2014: 73) that defy psychologized, behavioural approaches to lifestyle modification. Due to interviewees' relatively homogeneous backgrounds and the desirability to personalize their responses, pseudonyms are used throughout.

Healthism and perceptions of physical activity

Awareness of the clinically evaluated health benefits of taking part in regular physical activity was not only widespread but confused by a conflation of sport, exercise and other aspects of daily living. Some had received medical advice to stay active and 'not to give in to it' (Emily), others had proactively chosen to exercise to avoid the physical decline they saw in relatives, etc., who had respiratory and/or other illnesses, and some simply accepted the longstanding common-sense view embodied in the sport–health ideology; 'I mean intellectually you think well, if you were there doing an hour's PE every day it'd probably do you the world of good' (Neil). The notion that health consciousness was both fuelled and serviced by the expansion of the health product market (Crawford 2006) was evident in the extent that the corporations proactive in sponsoring PAHP policies (e.g. Nike, Technogym) benefited from these beliefs. Many catalogued their (often ultimately futile) economic outlay on exercise equipment designed to enable their attempts to become more physically active (treadmills exercise bikes, free weights, etc.).

People were largely wholly convinced that exercise 'makes you feel better', 'makes you feel better about yourself', and 'can be fun' (Jonas 2009: 5–6). Respondents recalled positive experiences of a wide range of activities, from attending the gym, dancing classes, playing golf and undertaking pulmonary rehabilitation. Frequently people equated activity with a perception of healthiness – 'When I was doing the exercises a year ago, I was doing well' (David) – ranging from weight loss to a more holistic feeling of well-being. As Samuel said, 'the more exercise you do the better I do feel absolutely ... the bit of exercise where I do get that heart pumping, afterwards I feel better. Mentally it definitely gives you a buzz'. For many though this intermingled with nostalgia, particularly reminiscences of physical education at school and country walks during adulthood. The link between activity and pleasure was particularly evident in the direct association people made between exercise and being on holiday: 'When we go on holiday we do a lot more walking and whether it's the sea air that helps me breathe [I don't know but] ... I'm a lot more active then' (Olivia).

But these views were also partly shaped by the health imperative (Lupton 1995) and the socially defined desirability of exercise. Respondents typically expressed the notion that health was something that was individually achieved stating, for instance, 'I've got to admit it's one of those things, I ought to make an effort' (Samuel). While some reflexively complained about the persistence of PAHP messages in the press, others demonstrated a remarkable degree of voluntary self-compulsion (Lupton 1995). For example, a man whose condition was so severe that he used an oxygen machine throughout the interview described the extent of his attempts to live 'healthily':

> Yes and I think the secret is, I mean I'll tell everybody this who I see struggling, the fitter you can keep yourself the better. Now in my case, I can't walk now; I can't walk very far anyway. That's my biggest

downfall. So [I use] the bike because I'm not carrying my body weight but I'm still getting exercise and that's the thing.

(Steve)

The penetration of medical paradigms into the identities and everyday lives of these individuals was very much apparent. Tellingly, Steve contrasts his own condition with those he thinks 'struggle' and thus projects himself as a successful self-manager of health (Timmermans 2013). One interviewee who had primarily expressed a chaos narrative and spoke very emotionally about her struggle for a diagnosis which reflected her subjectively experienced symptoms, explained:

I'll try and do it every day because I think, I know it's not far, but if I can just get down and get a newspaper every day, I'm still walking, I'm still keeping active, it is still some form of exercise. And it would be very easy, especially with not being able to do a lot of stuff at home, to just sit in the chair and just vegetate, and I don't want that.

(June)

It was evident therefore that public health agencies had been relatively successful in raising consciousness if nothing else.

Interviewees who presented themselves as effective self-managers of their condition (be it through a challenge, contrary or coping narrative), expressed a degree of pride in being physically active that correlates with a perception of virtuous citizenship. An interviewee who considered herself both currently active and physically fit explained how she always took the car, even for short trips, because, 'As I say, I think probably – you know, because I play golf and I do enough walking really' (Helen). The sense of moral worth was sufficient to be used to justify less compliant health behaviours on other occasions. For instance, another interviewee recalled how he had motivated himself to use an exercise bike:

I was getting quite into it you know just thinking crude rule of thumb it says you've burnt fifty calories – a load of cobblers – but just as a rule of thumb you say right a pint of Pedigree [beer] is 170 calories so if I ride the bike for a little. I got quite in the habit of it; it's ten minutes.

(Samuel)

But as Crawford (2006) suggests, healthism is accompanied by significant elements of victim-blaming of those who appear unwilling to conform to prescribed behaviours. This could be a source of frustration to some as they physically struggled to meet the expectations of others; 'I've had people say, "Oh you've got to get up and you've got to exercise. You've got to move about." Yeah you can, but not for long? A few minutes and that's it' (Emily). These experiences led some to project their compliance with PAHP messages in ways that avoided the potential stigma of being perceived as 'inactive'. The following extract is from an interview that was interrupted by the interviewee's partner walking into the living room:

DM: Would you normally walk to the shops or take the car?

MARK: Well, that depends on the sort of mood I'm in. [To partner] Don't laugh.

(All laugh)

PARTNER: *Do you want the truth?*

MARK: He takes the car usually.

PARTNER: *Yes.*

MARK: But sometimes I walk down.

PARTNER: *Very, very occasionally.*

DM: Is that convenience or is it because it's difficult to walk down or—?

MARK: No, not the walking down. It's the walking back that's the problem sometimes. I've got a poorly hip. It's not very good and it wants looking at. But I do walk down. I walk down and walk back up.

DM: Is it uphill, back?

MARK: Yes. Quite a good walk up the hill.

DM: Yes. You're not that near, are you?

MARK: Well, the shop's down the bottom. I think it's five-hundred yards from here down to the shops and five-hundred yards back. Yes, I lead a rather sedentary life I suppose you could say.

DM: Do you feel you ought to be more physically active?

MARK: Yes, definitely.

DM: What stops you?

MARK: I don't feel I ought to – I'm too lazy, I suppose.

These experiences illustrate the degree to which notions of healthism and the primary messages and social consequences of the NPH are experienced amongst the population. Exacerbated perhaps by the stigma associated with having an illness medically and social viewed as smoking-related (Lindqvist and Hallberg 2010), the virtuosity of physical activity in contemporary societies was engrained as part of the habitus of this cohort. Despite overwhelmingly 'buying in' to the health imperative and PAHP messages, the conceptual level medicalization was often counterbalanced at the interactional level by the problems encountered in the implementation of such 'good' intentions.

The barriers to physical activity

While some mentioned how their exercise opportunities were limited by structural constraints – such as being unable to gain access to PR programmes due to a lack of available places, or the lack of transport making it difficult to get to exercise-conducive environments out of the city – the primary concern was that exercise was rarely experienced as medicinal and, more frequently, as potentially health-harming. For instance, one interviewee said that they had given up swimming because, 'suddenly I got a bit panicky. I thought well I won't be able to take my oxygen' (Anthony). Another more explicitly rejected exercise because of the fear of the negative health consequences: 'I'm not going to kill myself … I'm not going to cripple myself going up and down the street and hurt myself more' (David). A third explained this ambiguity particularly clearly;

> I don't know in my own mind whether I'm doing myself harm or good. I know intellectually, I think this is great, I'd rather keep doing it as long as I can but I do get a lot of chest ache, and I don't know if sometimes I've overdone it a bit.
>
> (Neil)

Contrary to the messages exhorted in EiM therefore, exercise does not necessarily make people feel good and, in the case of underlying illness, can actually make people feel that they are exacerbating existing health problems.

In a similar vein, interviewees rarely spoke of exercise as helping them to 'feel younger' but noted, conversely, that they became conscious of their advancing age *specifically when they exercised*. People were conscious that they couldn't 'do as much now as I was doing then' and while some felt that exercise could help slow down the speed of their physical decline, the ageing process was experienced as both inevitable and irreversible. The embodied experience of illness was important in this:

> It hits me that I can't and it throws me. It seems to have put it in my sub-conscious, because in my head I feel as though I'm still a young person but my body's telling me now, 'Oy slow down, you're not how you think you are – 24 – you're 57, 58 now. Slow down. You can't do what you did then'.
>
> (Karl)

A common response indicative of an attempt to draw a compromise between the health imperative and the realities of physical activity, was to stress the value of being active, but 'in my own time and pace' (June). Interviewees described the importance of taking their time, knowing their limits, and doing 'what your body tells you to do' (Tom). Consequently people spoke about 'going to do what I can do, and that's it' (David), and rejecting the authority of medical advice in the belief that 'the best person to decide how much exercise I need is me not you' (Mike). Frequently, interviewees identified co-morbidities as a significant restriction on regular exercise participation. Typically, interviewees identified additional conditions (a 'poorly hip', suspected fractured vertebrae, arthritic knees) as either limiting their mobility or 'giving me an awful lot of problems and so each step was really painful' (Danny). They were frequently conscious of the negative impact that this might have on their COPD, one interviewee noting for instance, 'I do feel restricted and not just from the breathing. But if I can't do these things because of my physical skeleton, then I'm not doing my lungs any good. So I'm sort of fighting a battle both ways' (April). In contrast to the prescriptions of PAHP, this group very clearly perceived a risk to exercise that thus fundamentally restricted the degree that this 'medicine' structured their everyday activities.

Such experiences fuelled the prevention paradox; i.e. at a high level of generality it was accepted that exercise was beneficial but at the level of the individual it could be perceived to have little personal benefit. Consequently, lay interpretations of medical advice could be superseded by lay epidemiologies derived from personal experience. Interviewees complained that the development of injury led to exercise cessation. Asked why he had decided to stop playing football, one man said:

> I think it's more injuries that I'm picking up and it's taking longer for them to heal. And you think to yourself, there's going to be a day where I'm going to get tackled or I'm going to get hurt and I'm not going to recover from it.
>
> (Nick)

Moreover, the interviewee could not see a satisfactory alternative form of exercise with which to replace football (see discussion of Andrew *et al.* 2014 in the conclusion to Chapter 5). Others presented evidence for the futility of exercising for health purposes:

> you say going out for exercise and stuff like that. My brother, he did that, he went biking, him and his wife went biking, and he dropped dead of a heart attack last year. Fit as a fiddle, never been to the doctors, he just – you know. So there's a theory in it ... they're saying if you're fat and all the rest of it it's bad for you, you're going to die. But you're going to die anyway, aren't you really.
>
> (Mike)

Those not limited by concerns that exercise may be harmful to their health described motivations that resonate with the importance of a quest for exciting significance in leisure (Maguire 1992). Gyms in particular were identified as providing an unpleasant exercise experience, typically described as 'boring' (Neil, Danny, April). Others provided descriptions that resonated with a sense of exclusion from the environments populated by those who were 'fit for consumption' (Smith-Maguire 2008). For example, the gym environment was found to be 'anathema ... pretty horrifying' (Samuel) due to perceptions that one was 'surrounded by people looking in mirrors' (Danny).

Most commonly however, despite the recognition that it was conducive to improved health, interviewees rejected exercise as they simply did not find it served any 'purpose'. As one interviewee noted, 'I don't mind walking and stopping for a beer but I can't see the point of just going for a walk, just to admire things. What a waste of life' (Joe). Another who had tried exercising at home in an explicit attempt to improve health invoked nostalgia when trying to describe his antipathy towards such regimented exercise routines:

> I think it's just the – I find it a bit boring, do you know, and I'll get on a cycle machine and I find cycling in the bedroom, it was actually no fun at all. I used to enjoy cycling, going around the village lanes and things, so no [I don't do it anymore].
>
> (Neil)

That sense of purpose did not necessarily need to be particularly tangible but it did need to be meaningful to the individuals involved and ultimately this centred on pleasure. For instance one interviewee explained that, 'If I do exercise ... it's for a reason. If I do my exercise – walking – it's because I enjoy it' (April). For this cohort (lack of) enjoyment could be closely associated with their illness and the exacerbation of symptoms. The importance of finding an activity that engendered some form of meaning was identified by people who welcomed the physical challenge of, for instance, attempting to climb a hill, and was summarized by one man in particular who said, 'So really to a point if you're not happy doing what you're doing then why do it. Better to die happy I think than to die a sad man, you know what I mean?' (Fred). Thus, while exercise certainly *could* be fun, most of the time it was not, and when it was it was for reasons that had little to do with its health-promoting qualities. Here, PAHP is undone due to the elusive nature of 'fitness' within contemporary conceptions of health.

Finally, and in marked contrast to the idealized versions of exercise described in PAHP in Chapter 4, many experienced physical activity as fundamentally destructive to their broader social relations; that is to say, loneliness and a sense of social isolation are *exacerbated* by attempts to be physically active. For instance, exercising was frequently depicted as incompatible with the demands of both work productivity and family duties. As in previous studies, interviewees described themselves as too busy to exercise (Thorpe *et al.* 2012) and simply struggled to commit to an exercise routine alongside work. As one noted:

> It's just getting the willpower, the time together … by five o'clock I'm on my bloody knees mentally. I'll get in about an hour early just to try and get some peace and quiet, but at the moment the sheer onslaught of multiple things you just [can't manage].
>
> (Samuel)

Some ceased physical activity because of the impact it was having on work; 'Like I used to cycle to work, but then no, I don't cycle anymore. I'm too tired when I get to work to actually work, so I went in the car' (Jonathon). Others described the perception that devoting time to exercise could be perceived as 'selfish' and thus had to be sacrificed 'because I'm not neglecting family' (Anthony). A female who was the primary carer for her mother explained,

> my physical fitness has gone down because I'm going at my mum's pace all the time.… There's nothing anybody can do about it and by the time I get home I can't go to the gym, no way, I'm too shattered.
>
> (April)

For many, therefore, the decision (not) to exercise was never a 'discrete issue' (Prior *et al.* 2014: 73) but, rather, had to be viewed within a holistic understanding of the demands of contemporary living. Choosing to exercise was not a simple, individualistic choice but a complex and socially negotiated dilemma.

Indeed, ultimately, decisions about achievable physically activity levels entailed the resolution of a number of contradictory considerations. Some cited the unpredictability of the built environment (will there be lifts or stairs? will there be places to sit and rest?) and the weather ('I don't mind walking out in the rain – that's great for me – it's the heat' (Karl)), but those with more severe COPD may not be prepared to walk or exercise alone through fears of exacerbating their condition. As one interviewee explained, 'I won't go too far because I can get stressed and I can feel unwell' (Mike). However, attempts to exercise with family members could be equally if not more problematic:

> The thing that does frustrate me even with my grandchildren and that, if they take me out shopping or anywhere that's fine, but they walk a – I'll start off with a reasonable speed but then I get slower and slower so I start lagging behind. And my grandson will often say, 'Hang on wait for nanny, she's fallen behind again, don't rush off and leave her.'
>
> (Emily)

Indicative of the negative social experience of walking with family, this interviewee concluded, 'you feel you're a bit of a pest'.

Even when physical activity was simplified into a couples rather than group activity, problems could still occur. Some noted that 'I mean I can't walk at my wife's pace. She slows down to walk at my pace now' (Neil), while conversely others noted that their partners would urge them to slow down, saying, ' "I need to keep up with you. You need to slow down a bit" ' (April). This was significant enough to deter some couples from going for a walk together – 'The wife often says she's going to [go for a walk] then when I suggest it she doesn't want to. So we don't bother' (Fred). It could even lead to overt conflict in partnerships:

> Now my husband wants to race on and he'll say, 'Oh you've only got to go this far' but I can't, my body is stopping me in my tracks. You can't do it, get your breath back first and then carry on. He understands a lot more now but in the past it used to almost cause rows.
>
> (Emily)

Not uncommonly, people curtailed their physical activities in order to safeguard the social relations that were important to them.

Conclusion

The lived reality of using exercise as a form of medicine is far more problematic and far more complex than is normally portrayed in the hypothetical scenarios contained in the policies extolling the medicalization of exercise. For many, taking part in exercise can deliver on the promise to 'make you feel better' and, if largely only nostalgically, is considered fun. But while the ubiquity of the sport–health ideology is fundamentally untouched in this process, EiM and other PAHP documents fundamentally simplify the choices individuals need to make, and the physical, environmental and social constraints that can potentially be faced.

More broadly, the sociology of health and illness literature suggests that patients tend to evaluate treatment programmes according to five central criteria: symptom relief; the degree to which they facilitate patient independence; the potential health risks and side-effects; the degree of time, difficulty and constraint involved; and the degree of embarrassment and stigma experienced (Williams 1993). In contrast, clinicians are predominantly only concerned with the first three. Thus, while exercise might be biomedically evaluated as reducing breathlessness, enhancing quality of life and posing relatively few negative side-effects (though these, as we have seen, may be underestimated), the lived experience can be markedly different. For those diagnosed with COPD, exercise appears, in the short-term at least, to exacerbate rather than ease physical discomfort, present logistical problems in terms of finding suitable activities and environments and increase dependence on, if not lead to conflict with, significant others.

Exercise may entail multiple and contradictory forms of embarrassment and stigma – from the public display of unpleasant symptoms (coughing) to the sense of deviance in struggling or failing to conform to public health messages. In many respects COPD patients reject exercise as medicine exactly because they are rational consumers of healthcare and not because they are misguided in their choices (Lupton 1995). Moreover, the stigma that can be generated from a sense of non-compliance may create iatrogenic outcomes in the form of perceptions of guilt. The promise of EiM, that exercise will make you 'feel better about yourself', becomes a self-fulfilling prophecy; the sense of well-being could simply (or partly) be a manifestation of the social morality of exercising.

In conclusion therefore, we can see that while there is broad acceptance of the medicalization of sport (and exercise) at the conceptual level, this does not have a more enduring social impact due to the problems of implementation at the interactional level. As much as the surveillance component of PAHP reaches out into the identities and dominates citizens' knowledge and understanding of the medicinal aspects of exercise, medical dominance is resisted at the interactional level due to the complexity of embodied experiences and the social interdependencies in which individuals are enmeshed. For a significant proportion of the public therefore, medicalization fundamentally affects their thinking but not necessarily their actions.

* * *

We return to these issues in the conclusion of this book (Chapter 11) but next we turn our attention to the more longstanding and traditional domain of sports medicine, namely the supply of medical services to the elite sport population. We begin by looking at the provision of sports medicine and healthcare in a range of professional and representative sports, seeking to assess sports medicine as it is provided as a form of occupational medicine. Second, we examine the practice of medicine in sport and specifically the degree to which the context, clients and co-workers curtail medical dominance in this particular practice setting. Finally we focus on two specific issues – concussion and cardiac screening – to provide more focused illustrations of the dynamics of figurations in which the traditions and cultures of sport come into conflict with the desires and demands of (sports) medicine.

Chapter 7

Sports medicine as occupational medicine

As we saw in Chapter 3, the institutional emergence of sports medicine has largely been a messy and incoherent process. This belies the dominant narrative that, over the course of the twentieth century, the pursuit of competitive success in elite sport not only led to the more extensive use, but also the increasingly systematic and rational exploitation, of medical science (Hoberman 1992). This argument implies a particular sort of medicalization: an expansion of the scope of practice driven by external evaluations of medicine's esoteric skills, in which the medical profession is reactive and accommodating rather than imperialistic (de Swaan 1989). This chapter builds on that analysis by exploring a 'who', 'what' and 'why' of medical provision in performance, professional or commercial sport. Specifically, in this chapter we examine who it is that works in the field, what kind of medical cover is provided, and why, or to what degree, has the pursuit of athletic excellence shaped this provision? The conclusion drawn from a comparison of a range of existing studies is that economic exigencies, institutional idiosyncrasies and patient preference has meant that medicine's jurisdictional expansion into elite sport has been somewhat exaggerated in the literature. More accurately such developments are symptomatic of the rather stilted 'professionalization' of the sub-discipline more generally. In this respect the medicalization of sport has been partial and piecemeal.

A typology of occupational healthcare

In contrast to previous discussions of definitional difficulties regarding sports medicine (see Chapter 3), the necessarily narrower field of professional sport entails a relatively coherent body of medical provision, for if we focus on the healthcare provided by sports teams and NGBs it is reasonable to conceive of sports medicine as a form of occupational healthcare. This is one area of sports medicine that can meaningfully be defined by patient demographics.

In this respect Kotarba (2001) argues that different types of occupational medicine can be distinguished in relation to their organizational structure and working culture. Structurally, 'the quality and complexity of occupational health care is a function of the relative value of the work to the employer' (Kotarba 2001: 767). Consequently, the most highly valued employees receive individualized and preventative healthcare (e.g. lifestyle management, health club membership, etc.), while the lowest merely have access to periodic screening and health assessments designed to ensure a person possesses the necessary physical capacity to carry out the expected duties. The work culture, however, is seen to dictate the 'style, tone and meaning of occupational health care delivery' (Kotarba 2001: 767). Occupational medicine does not simply attend to the physiological needs of workers, but is more broadly shaped by the norms of the workplace subculture, e.g. the emphasis on optimal, advanced and ground-breaking performance as opposed to routine and quantifiable productivity.

On this basis Kotarba (2001) identifies three main types of occupational healthcare. *Elite* occupational healthcare is the most medically advanced available and potentially the most expensive. Culturally, it is highly individualized such that the worker is seen as a patient-client who makes an irreplaceable contribution to workplace productivity. Typically, elite occupational healthcare is deemed to be complex and is thus provided by a medical practitioner who specializes in the field. *Managed* occupational healthcare is provided to workers who are not deemed to be particularly special and could be replaced relatively easily. Culturally, it will reflect this rationale, concerned to balance the expense of delivery against the savings accrued from having a healthy workforce. Typically, managed occupational healthcare is provided by a medical generalist (e.g. a GP) who works for, and reports to, the organization rather than the individual. Finally, *Primitive* occupational medicine is made available to the least valuable, most easily replaced and low-skilled workers. Culturally, healthcare is seen as benevolence or charity. There is no pretence to health optimization, just a desire to 'patch up the worker in an incidental manner – when care is available and when there is an immediate need for care' (Kotarba 2001: 768). For these reasons, primitive occupational healthcare is typically delivered by an ancillary health worker, such as a nurse or physiotherapist. Applying this tripartite model to American sports medicine, Kotarba suggests that elite occupational healthcare is available to the leading performers in individual sports such as golf and tennis and those in major league team sports (NBA, NFL, etc.); managed healthcare is the norm within less wealthy team sports (e.g. American men's soccer leagues and the women's NBA); and semi-professional or amateur sports performers only have access to primitive care.

Two key issues arise from Kotarba's (2001) model. First, each form of occupational healthcare suggests notions of medical power that falls some way short of the traditional conceptions of medical professionalism which underpin the medicalization thesis. In particular, the importance of economic interests in this model provides direct parallels with Johnson's (1972) Marxist-oriented analysis of professions. Elite occupational healthcare is similar to what Johnson describes as the patronage model, in which (medical) consumers define both their own needs and the manner in which those needs are served, ultimately leading the (healthcare) professional to become the 'client'. Managed occupational healthcare (and to a lesser extent Primitive) is similar to Johnson's definition of the mediative model, in which a third party (here the sports organization) arbitrates between (medical) producer and (athlete–patient) consumer, assessing the validity of consumers' needs and the manner in which the producer will attend to those needs. No model of occupational healthcare defined by Kotarba matches what Johnson describes as the classic form of professionalism, the collegiate model, in which the producer defines the needs of the consumer and the manner in which these needs are served. Suffice to say, occupational healthcare may represent medicalization in the sense of jurisdictional expansion, but medicalization that is neither driven by nor enhances the autonomy of the profession. Second, if the 'medicalization through rational pursuit of athletic success' hypothesis is correct, sports medicine would: (a) increasingly come to resemble elite occupational healthcare; (b) be most advanced in the most commercial sports; and (c) develop concomitantly with the intensification of commercialization processes.

This chapter uses Kotarba's hierarchy of occupational medicine to evaluate studies of the medical and healthcare provision in sport. Initially, we examine studies of primitive occupational healthcare in sport, augmenting Kotarba's US-based research with other American, Canadian and British studies. Subsequently, we explore models of managed occupational healthcare, focusing on medical provision in the wealthiest sport in England (football), and under conditions of heightened financial investment in post-professional rugby union. Third, we explore evidence for the existence of elite occupational healthcare, charting the provision for Olympic athletes in both Britain and Canada. As we will see, the empirical evidence demonstrates that while primitive occupational healthcare clearly exists in amateur and semi-professional sport, Kotarba's belief in the existence of elite and/or managed occupational healthcare in professional sport is largely a matter of conjecture. We conclude by drawing on studies of the integration of medicine and science in sport, which provides a segue into the subsequent chapter focusing on the everyday practice of sports medicine. Ultimately, though, the absence of elite occupational healthcare in sport highlights the peculiar dynamics of the medicalization of sport, largely determined by people within the world of sport rather than medicine and, in particular, structured according to the cultural norms of the former.

Primitive occupational healthcare in sport

Kotarba's (2001) study of rodeo riders and wrestlers provides the most detailed account of primitive occupational healthcare. Although prize money in professional rodeo amounts to millions of dollars per year, participants frequently have to pay an entrance fee and, as their earnings may not cover the high travel expenses of their nomadic lifestyles, many seek part-time work, primarily of a manual nature. Injuries to riders are common and expected (Kotarba cites one study that found that 14% of participants were injured in a single day), but they are also integrated into the dramatic spectacle. The healthcare provided through the Justin Sportsmedicine Program (sponsored by the Justin cowboy boot company) is essentially charitable and in large part a public relations exercise for the organizers. The 'Justin heelers' (heeling being a pun on the term for calf roping) are usually athletic trainers who are experienced in the nature of rodeo injuries and the behaviour of livestock.[1] They embrace the rodeo lifestyle, dressing and acting like their 'patients'. They treat large numbers of riders (approximately 70 per rodeo) and thus provide (in a phrase that evokes the medical provision at large civic marathons, see Chapter 1) 'battlefield-type healthcare' with an emphasis on enabling the rider's participation as they 'patch him up as best they can' (Kotarba 2001: 773). Local professional wrestling provides a similarly precarious occupation, attracting audiences of a couple of hundred and paying participants a few hundred dollars per fight. Wrestlers therefore frequently engage in additional paid work (many are also college students) and are drawn to wrestling by the identity validating experience of physical contact; 'they love to hit and be hit' (Kotarba 2001: 774). As in rodeo, injury rates are high but here participants sign contracts that waive promoters' health-related liability. Consequently, wrestlers might source medical aid through their work-related insurance (although such policies will rarely cover sport-related injury, leading claimants into deceitful practices), through their parents' health insurance (if young enough) or with out-of-pocket payments for emergency medical treatment. A final option is the healthcare provided by the promoter. This is typically a free service offered by a former wrestler or wrestling administrator who also happens to have some healthcare experience (e.g. a physical or athletic therapist). This 'charitable' healthcare serves as a useful public relations function but is also frequently integrated into the spectacle of the wrestling. Kotarba concludes that in the 'marginal' professional sports of rodeo and wrestling, where athletes are lowly rewarded, easily replaced and have largely lower class occupational and educational backgrounds, 'the most prominent healthcare workers ... share in the athlete's culture and shape the actual delivery of healthcare accordingly' (Kotarba 2001: 777). The role of medicine is perhaps as much about placating audience expectations as it is about providing meaningful healthcare to participants.

Kotarba's (2012) subsequent study of healthcare provision in elite women's sport focuses on the Houston Pinks women's (American) football team. Rather than receive payment, team members are required to raise sponsorship of $1000 per season to cover travel costs. Kotarba illustrates how in this context healthcare is essentially ad hoc, voluntary or community based. For example, it was only through the coach's personal contacts (as a former NFL player) that the Pinks gained access to a training facility that had on-site physical therapists and athletic trainers. While league rules required teams to provide paramedical care for matches, there was none for training and, in emergency cases, players would simply have to drive their injured teammates to hospital. A doctor provided pro-bono cover at matches but there was no insurance to provide ongoing treatment. If players could draw on their own policies (again rare or fraudulent) they would be seen by their own doctor. Consequently, in the absence of more formal or centrally provided support, the team operated with a strong community healthcare ethos. This meant that players took responsibility for monitoring and controlling each other's well-being, would share lay medical knowledge and draw on the skills of teammates with healthcare training, and enjoy the support of a number of medically trained volunteers who attended games as spectators. Players who suffered severe injuries – the example of an ACL injury is cited – would simply have to remove themselves from the team while they recovered.

In contrast to Kotarba's assessment of the variations in occupational healthcare at different levels of sport, there is good reason to think that the primitive form is the norm in this field. The key evidence for this is the dependence – throughout sport – on ancillary healthcare workers rather than either generalists or specialists. For instance, referring to Britain, McEwen and Taylor (2010: 85) argue that 'even within professional sport, [physiotherapists] are often viewed as the dominant clinician', while Malcolm (2006a: 388) argues that 'physiotherapists do not simply assist doctors, but in many cases display considerable autonomy'. Similarly, in relation to Canada, Theberge (2009a: 267–68) notes that in both college and university athletic programmes, as well as 'professional sport teams ... athletic therapists (or trainers) are the primary providers of site coverage of athletic events, including immediate care for injuries'. Walk (2004: 257) agrees, noting that although athletic therapists in the US often nominally work under the supervision of a physician, 'generally, the athletic training programme in university sports is under the direction of a head athletic trainer'. Indeed, there have been a number of press exposés of healthcare provision in the NCAA (Walk 2004) and in part this must also relate to the reliance on Student Athletic Trainers who, by definition, are not fully trained yet deemed sufficiently senior to hold 'the authority to decide when athletes were ready to return to play' (Walk 1997: 36). Pike (2005) found that rowing clubs in England frequently did not offer any healthcare provision and, as a consequence of widespread perceptions of the incompetence and disinterest of family doctors, depended largely on CAMs. It also appears that female athletes are markedly less well catered for than their male counterparts (Kotarba 2012; Theberge 2000). Thus, overall, in structure, culture and particularly personnel deployed, studies consistently depict occupational healthcare in sport that essentially exhibits the characteristics of what Kotarba describes as primitive provision (further evidence of the widespread nature of primitive healthcare in sport is described in Chapter 8).

Managed occupational healthcare in sport

Rob Huizenga's *You're Okay, It's Just a Bruise* (1995, cited in Waddington 2012), is the autobiographical account of the team physician for the NFL's Los Angeles Raiders between 1983 and 1990. Huizinga notes that his interview for the post consisted of three questions about his own sporting participation, one about his college education, and finally the enquiry, 'have you ever played hurt?' Huizinga's account reveals how interference by the club owner led to a range of questionable medical practices, including: the prescription of anabolic steroids; being instructed by the owner to misrepresent or not disclose information about players' injuries; and denying appropriate medical provision to a player with a neck injury because the club owner felt that, 'the team get demoralised and plays less aggressively when they see a teammate getting carted off the field on a stretcher' (Huizenga 1995, cited in Waddington 2012: 209). Huizenga noted that he was paid an annual salary that was less than most players received per game.

What Huizenga describes is essentially managed occupational healthcare. There was little concern to attract a medical specialist, the expenditure was low especially relative to other salaries in the workplace, worker-athletes were treated as fundamentally replaceable and high levels of managerial control were exerted over healthcare providers. This account defies Kotarba's hypothesis in that it depicts managed rather than elite occupational healthcare in American major league sport. One could perhaps argue that the atypicality of this kind of exposé, the commercial incentive to sensationalize particular themes in a text such as this and the now dated account should lead us to be cautious in generalizing these findings. But evidence from sports settings in the UK, where like the NFL Kotarba would predict the existence of elite occupational healthcare, contains many parallels. Shortly we will examine healthcare provision in rugby union but first we turn our attention to the medical provision in the most commercial and affluent British sport, football. Once again, this shows limited evidence that medicine has deeply penetrated sport or is being rationally applied in the relentless pursuit of physical excellence.

Healthcare provision in English professional football

Professional football is not only the sport with the longest tradition of providing occupational healthcare, but incorporates the most highly paid and famous athletes in England. However, as Carter (2009b: 70) argues, the development of the football club doctor role has historically been shaped not by economic rationality but by commitments to the amateur ethos in sport and 'a tradition of voluntarism that was not only deep-rooted in medicine but also in British society'. Football club doctors were invariably GPs, acquired their position through personal contacts and were rarely paid (Carter 2009b cites a 1961–1962 survey which showed that just 13 of 45 respondents received financial remuneration). Their motivations, rather, were based on cultural expectations that they would contribute to civic culture, and also interpersonal rewards such as the opportunity to mix with the social elite and the consequent raised profile and social status of the individual. Many were even appointed onto the executive boards of football clubs in recognition of their service. As we have seen (see Chapter 3), in line with this, many football club doctors were disconnected from the sports medicine profession (Carter 2009b). Frequently though, it was the football trainer who performed the primary role in injury treatment. Trainers were usually former players and in that their methods were largely experientially developed and orally transmitted, were similar to 'alternative-unorthodox practitioners like bone setters, herbalists and osteopaths' (Carter 2009a: 262). Despite these traditions, Carter (2007: 417) believes that, 'greater financial risks and fiercer competition has seen sports medicine become an increasingly important aspect of the preparation of players'. To what extent has this most lucrative and wealthy branch of sport become medicalized through the rational exploitation of science?

Research at the turn of the millennium suggested that the answer to this question was 'not much'. Waddington et al. (2001) used questionnaires and qualitative interviews to study doctors, physiotherapists and current and retired players in English professional football. They argued that club doctors rarely had specialist sports medicine qualifications, relevant occupational experience or formal contracts, and that they agreed to provide essentially charitable work (either unpaid or compensated well below BMA recommended rates) simply because, in many cases, they were fans of the team. Most spent relatively little time at the football club or attending to players. Only in the highest leagues did clubs devote the necessary economic resources to ensure that they had their own doctor available at both home and away fixtures.

The traditional dominance of the football trainer was therefore enduring. Moreover, the research revealed that just half of all 'physiotherapists' were chartered, and that many were ex-footballers who held only the Football Association (FA) Diploma in the Treatment of Injuries and so were not sufficiently qualified to practice in the British NHS. Many physiotherapists had no other medical occupational experience and were directly dependent on a personal relationship with the football club manager for their employment. The authors argued that selection and appointment procedures represented a 'catalogue of poor employment practice' (Waddington et al. 2001: 51), and that under these conditions it was difficult for healthcare workers to resist threats to their clinical autonomy and/or to maintain ethical standards (parallels can be drawn with employment conditions and practice norms in the NFL as described by Huizenga. The implications for sports medicine practice are discussed in Chapter 8).

The conditions described in English professional football at this time belie the assumption that significant financial resources necessarily entail the development of elite occupational healthcare. Provision most closely resembled Kotarba's (2001) definition of managed or, in many cases, primitive occupational healthcare. Football club medicine was either structurally dependent on individual benevolence or was provided at very limited cost. Healthcare was delivered either by a generalist or, frequently, an ancillary worker. Perhaps more significant than economic factors in structuring the organization of sports medicine, was the sub-cultural conventions of professional sport. As Waddington (2002: 62) noted, 'the standards of care with which they [football club physiotherapists] will be familiar will not be the clinical and ethical standards of care which apply within the health service, but rather those which derive from the culture of football'.

Recommendations derived from this research (Waddington et al. 2001) and the subsequent press and medical-professional reaction (Boyce 2001; Mackay 2001) moved the FA to revise its medical regulations. These currently state that: all club doctors (appointed post-2003) require a specialist sports medicine qualification; all senior club physiotherapists should be chartered (although exceptionally clubs may employ a graduate sports therapist); and that medical staff must undergo specified levels of continuous professional development (FA 2015).[2] However, a subsequent survey undertaken in 2014 showed that while football club medical provision had become more extensive and increasingly professional over the intervening 15-year period, significant elements of managed occupational healthcare remained (see Appendix for an outline of the research method).

While we do not have directly comparable data from the earlier survey, it seems clear that clubs have, as the medicalization and rationalization of sport thesis would suggest, come to more fully exploit the promise of medicine and sports science. Clubs employed up to seven doctors (mean = 2.33), eight physiotherapists (mean = 3.7) and 10 'other' healthcare providers (mean = 2.94) with, as might be expected, the size of MDTs (multidisciplinary teams) roughly concordant with clubs' divisional status, competitive success, wealth, etc. Moreover, it was clear that significant improvements in relation to the qualifications and experience of both club doctors and physiotherapists had been made. Most club doctors were still GPs (64%) but many now had specialist qualifications in sports medicine (63%) and relevant occupational experience (30% had worked in multiple football clubs, 33% in multiple sports). While only a third travelled to away fixtures and the marked increase in the number of hours doctors assigned to football club work suggested that increasing amounts of time were spent providing ongoing treatment to players rather than mandatory emergency cover. While the earlier study found that frequently the club doctor was a 'one-sport, one-club doctor' and that their 'commitment is typically not to sports medicine in general but to their local club' (Waddington 2002: 58), increasingly club doctors found a career path in sports medicine, with formal contracts more frequently held (44%), higher levels of payment, and more positions in football providing doctors with their primary employment (18%). For physiotherapists, reliance on the FA Diploma for the Treatment of Injuries was a historical relic and approximately a quarter of physiotherapists even had a relevant postgraduate qualification. Physiotherapists experienced greater job security (62% had been in post for over three years) suggesting a greater degree of autonomy from individual managers (their average tenure being less than 18 months). Evidence suggested, however, that the transparency (advertising posts) and rigour (interviewing candidates) of the appointment process still fell short of employment best practice (see also Wagstaff *et al.* 2015).

Thus, medical provision in professional English football had diversified from a mixture of managed and primitive occupational healthcare to span all three levels of Kotarba's typology. An interview with a physiotherapist at one of the richest Premiership clubs revealed how comprehensive this elite healthcare provision could be. The physiotherapist had a postgraduate qualification, relevant occupational experience and was specializing in sports practice when they responded to an advert in the *Physiotherapy Journal*. Prior to appointment they had two interviews with a panel containing the existing physiotherapist, club doctor, manager, a club director and the club secretary. Over time the original team of three physiotherapists had grown to eight full-time plus some additional, casual or part-time appointments, and the club had a full-time director of medical services, a full-time doctor and an academy doctor contracted for 16 hours per week. The club had enabled physiotherapists to undertake postgraduate qualifications (both financially and through day release), had a strong Continuing Professional Development (CPD) programme including internal training, and conducted annual and quadrennial audits in which provision was evaluated by a university professor of physiotherapy. The club physiotherapist described a highly individualized healthcare system with each player assigned a personal clinical lead, requests for specialist treatment outside of the club were tolerated and sometimes club-funded, and systematically collected player feedback influencing overall provision. In sum, it was believed that treatment 'should be patient-led, so if the patient is happy somewhere else because the philosophy fits in to what they've been brought up on, then that's fine and we're happy for them to go there' (Premiership physiotherapist).

However, the process of medicalization evident in these findings needs to be tempered by an acknowledgement of both the limited rationality behind, and reach of, these processes. First, it is remarkable that whilst many more opportunities to gain a sports medicine qualification now exist (see Chapter 3), over a third of football club doctors still do not have specialist qualifications. That football clubs continue to employ non-specialists, at times in contravention of FA regulations (two questionnaire respondents did not have a SEM qualification, had been appointed post-2003, had no previous professional football club experience and were therefore in contravention of FA regulations), illustrates continued disregard for the value of sport-specific medical expertise. Second, the reluctance of (most) clubs to financially invest in occupational healthcare was reiterated by the findings that only 60% of current club doctors received a salary and that some healthcare providers identified levels of CPD that seemed to fall below FA-stipulated thresholds. That only about a quarter of all club doctors were appointed after an interview conducted by someone qualified to assess their medical expertise, suggests that the prevalent view within English professional football was that healthcare requirements were neither especially advanced nor complex, and that cost remained a central consideration. Elite occupational healthcare may, therefore, exist in the very highest echelons of the most commercially-lucrative sport in Britain, but more frequently we see managed occupational healthcare and in some cases stronger evidence of a primitive system. For instance, a GP who was doctor at a lower league club described the very limited role they saw for themselves:

> I'm not kind of a sports specialist. I've got no sports qualifications. We're dealing with professional sports people so I very much make it my aim to not give opinions on sporting injuries ... if they have a problem, you know kind of an injury, then I leave that to the physios.

Healthcare provision in English professional rugby union

While the example of football illustrates the (limited) impact that a wealth of resources can have on medical provision, examination of the healthcare provision in rugby union provides an apposite illustration of the impact of commercialization-led policy change. In 1995, rugby union relinquished its amateur tradition and allowed aspects of professionalism into the game. In

England specifically, the post-1995 'open' era was marked by: the (overt) payment of players; the organizational re-structuring of clubs including expanded playing and support staffs; rule changes to create a more dynamic game; and fixture re-packaging and re-scheduling to generate greater spectator appeal (Malcolm *et al.* 2000). A 2000–2001 survey of the management of injuries at the top 68 rugby clubs in the country (see Appendix) came in the midst of a relatively late and rapid phase of commercialization.

In some respects, findings mirrored the situation revealed in professional football (Malcolm 2006a; Malcolm and Sheard 2002). Few club doctors self-identified as sports-specialists, had specialist qualifications or sport-specific occupational experience. Rather, most were GPs, recruited and appointed informally and receiving little or no remuneration (some even claimed to subsidize the club by supplying strappings, etc.). They volunteered a relatively small amount of time due to a sense of civic duty, a love of the game and its social aspects, and sometimes the kudos associated with the role. In contrast to football, however, physiotherapists in rugby were formally contracted, career-oriented, sports-specialists. They typically had relevant qualifications and/or occupational experience, received (in their eyes) reasonable financial remuneration for working full time, and cited occupational experience as an important motivation. As a doctor with a leading team noted:

> The physiotherapists ... from what I've seen are absolutely stunning. They are very, very, very focused and very well qualified. They are very sports specific. They don't want to deal with normal physio problems like back pain, swollen joints, old geriatrics.... They want to deal with the sharp end.
>
> (Cited in Malcolm 2006a: 388)

Not surprisingly, the research revealed significant differences in provision across the hierarchy of leagues and clubs' respective financial resources, but a central conclusion was, 'that whilst medical cover for players is both quantitatively and qualitatively limited, the treatment of players' injuries has dramatically improved as a result of the professionalization of the game' (Malcolm and Sheard 2002: 158; see also Howe 2001). Commercial developments had invoked more formal appointment processes, standardized contractual arrangements, and undermined the dominance of the honorary/ volunteer club doctor. With professionalism, many doctors had introduced mid-week injury assessment clinics and many were now funded to travel to away matches. As a doctor with a leading side noted, 'All the teams now that we're professional bring a doctor with them.... It used to be the case that they didn't – 5 years ago – and it's all changed' (cited in Malcolm and Sheard 2002: 158). Professionalism had also led to the introduction of full-time physiotherapists (where players were full-time) and the employment of multiple physiotherapists at individual clubs. This meant that there was always medical provision at training and that, rather than players self-sourcing healthcare as they had done in the past, clubs could offer more continuous treatment and operate greater control over players' rehabilitation. Interviewees described the greater willingness of clubs to bear the cost of the referral of players to specialist medical services, and elements of innovative and experimental practice as medical provision became more flexible and more closely tailored to the individual. For instance, one player argued that, 'at the professional side of things, the clubs are taking a lot more care of the players. Medical staff; there seems to be more around and around more often' (cited in Malcolm and Sheard 2002: 155).

Again it is important not to overstate the quality of this medical provision – even in the best case scenarios, the descriptions exhibited the characteristics of Kotarba's managed occupational healthcare – or extrapolate too widely from accounts of the most comprehensive provision within rugby. For present purposes the most salient point is that the medicalization and commercialization of sport can be two essentially interdependent social processes. Medical support in rugby was starting from a very low and particularly primitive base in the 'pre-professional' game and the most radical changes impacted on only a small number of clubs. Moreover, even if the impact of commercialization had been to raise awareness of the role of players as assets, the reliance on ancillary workers (physiotherapists) still suggested that athletes' health was not particularly highly valued. These processes illustrated the expansion of medicalization in the sense that a medical framework increasingly came to structure the understanding of how elite level performance should be developed, but not in the sense of the medical profession becoming centrally placed in the resolution of perceived social problems. We will return to these ideas in the conclusion, but next we explore the medical provision for Olympic athletes in our search for elite occupational medicine within the sports context.

Elite occupational healthcare: provision for British Olympic athletes

As noted in Chapter 3, hosting the London 2012 Olympics added significant impetus to the professional project of British sports medicine, accompanying its state recognition as a medical subdiscipline and adding a considerable increase in funding to the ongoing formalization and development of specialist educational qualifications. Concurrently, sports physiotherapy underwent considerable structural change. The Association of Chartered Physiotherapists in Sports Medicine (ACPSM) (founded in 1972 as a clinical interest group within the Chartered Society of Physiotherapy) developed a three-tier membership largely based on differences in CPD training. Developed partly as a regulatory requirement of the HPC, the ACPSM explicitly sought to respond to the increased demand for elite sport healthcare, and move away from a reliance upon sports physiotherapists who were perceived to work in sport as a 'hobby' (see Malcolm and Scott 2011: 515). Building on the ACPSM accreditation process, in the run up to London 2012, the BOA introduced an Elite Sport Register. Consequently, postgraduate qualifications, relevant work experience and references provided by clinicians and elite sport representatives were rewarded in a programme designed to 'demonstrate that members are committed to professional excellence' (BOA, 2006).

Research conducted in 2008/09 aspired to capture the degree to which these policy and organizational developments impacted on clinical provision and practice (Scott 2010; see also Appendix). Again in some respects the findings replicate those presented in relation to football and rugby union. A questionnaire and interview survey of lead doctors for the 35 Olympic sports found that many doctors were part-time GPs, appointed via informal procedures, receiving low levels of remuneration and often seeing athletes only on an irregular basis. Reflecting the institutional development of sports medicine more broadly, many did though have sports-specialist qualifications (76%). Parallel research with Olympic sport physiotherapists found that while appointments were frequently informal, most were relatively well-qualified (particularly through CPD), payment was the norm (but often relatively low) and contact with athletes was continuous but far from comprehensive. Notably, these findings mirror Theberge's (2009b) study of healthcare provision for Canadian Olympic athletes. Theberge found that most doctors and physiotherapists had specialist qualifications and were CASM-aligned and sports medicine career-minded. A minority were full-time sports specialists, combining their unpaid voluntary roles for the Canadian Olympic Committee/Canadian Sports Centre with other forms of sports medicine practice.

However, it also became clear that policy initiatives affecting British sports medicine had created divisions between those that were referred to as 'national governing body' (NGB) doctors/physiotherapists (71% and 50% of respondents respectively) and those contracted to the HCIS (Scott, A. 2012). The latter generally had higher qualifications, were more transparently and rigorously appointed and consequently had a more structured career pathway with written job descriptions, good financial rewards and greater job security. They frequently also saw athletes on a daily basis and were integrated into a wider network of sports medicine professionals. HCIS doctors expressed both their distinction from their NGB counterparts and an identity that embodied 'new professionalism'; part of a recognized network, clinically competent and up-to-date (evident through new qualifications), patient-centred and collaborative across disciplines (Jones and Green 2006). In describing themselves as 'specialist specialists', they juxtaposed their heightened 'sense of legitimacy and social status', with 'non-specialist' NGB doctors who were becoming increasingly marginalized from the new mainstream and whose claims to expert status were increasingly difficult to justify (Scott, A. 2012). The development of hierarchies within the two professions was, however, treated in opposing manners, as academicization was unequivocally welcomed within the medical sub-discipline, but treated ambivalently within physiotherapy. While many physiotherapists did recognize that engagement with CPD in particular helped develop the skill set of their profession and create 'career portfolios' (Scott. A. 2012: 583), they also questioned the clinical usefulness of formal qualifications and more closely equated expertise with commitment and experience. Here, then, medical provision came to resemble elite occupational healthcare as described by Kotarba. It was (relatively) expensive, specialist and individualized, if mainly only available in the larger, better funded, and more 'podium-prolific' Olympic sports.

Conclusion

Given the largely contradictory empirical evidence, Kotarba's depiction of the provision of different types/levels of occupational medicine in sport is largely based on the logic that economic forces will inevitably predominate over the social – that the assessment of the production value of the worker will override the norms of the subculture – and, by implication, that the medicalization of sport represents a rational and proportionate use of resources. As illustrated throughout this chapter, and explored in more detail in Chapters 8 and 9, neither necessarily applies. Before we move on to examine the nature of sports medicine practice in more detail, and the role that everyday work settings (Freidson 1970) have in structuring the knowledge, understanding and actions of sports clinicians, we explore the factors that 'restrict' healthcare provision even in the most well-funded, competitively elite, sports settings. These factors are both macro- and micro-oriented, structural and interpersonal. They suggest a mediative model of medical professionalism (Johnson 1972), with medical dominance challenged by complex, highly bureaucratized organizations, stringent managerial monitoring of medical practice and outcomes and thus relatively limited professional autonomy.

Despite budgets enhanced by the desire for international sporting success and national prestige, organizational resources for Olympic athletes are inevitably stretched. This is, perhaps, an inherent feature of Western states which, in contrast to the centralization of nations such as China (or the communist countries of Cold War Eastern Europe), accommodate geographically dispersed athletes. As Kerr (2012: 4) notes, countries such as New Zealand 'adopt a neoliberal model that does not contain a clear pathway for athletes and coaches to work with sports scientists'. Similarly, in Canada, administrators note the regional inconsistencies of their systems and stress the difficulties of coordinating different parts of a national support system (Theberge 2012). Such systems are further undermined by athletes' access to healthcare provision outside the network, ironically fuelled by the tendency for healthcare professions to reward members for undertaking voluntary work to build up a portfolio of practical experience. Further logistical difficulties include the disjointed nature of provision whereby, for instance, an athlete might undergo surgery but then fail to access the physiotherapy and strength and conditioning support required to return them to elite competition. Fundamentally, any occupational healthcare provision that is dependent on embodied performance for inclusion is prone to inefficiencies. The system of 'carding' in which 'podium potential' rather than medical need determines access to healthcare (Bundon and Clarke 2014; Theberge 2012) is likely to lead to Catch-22 situations where the injured (and therefore non-performing) athlete is deprived of the funding/medical support required to recover from injury. Athletes and coaches view the performance monitoring embedded in carding systems as both unreflective of, and a hindrance to, the development of athletic success (Kerr 2012).

Closely related to budgetary restrictions are variations in provision across performance and preparation sites. Differences are apparent in a comparison of healthcare support at major games (such as the Olympics) with that for training camps and minor competitions. Provision at major games is marked by the 'presence of a well-equipped medical clinic staffed by a multidisciplinary team of healthcare professionals' (Theberge 2009b: 53). While clinicians are time-pressured, this fosters inter-professional collaboration, with the healthcare that athletes receive driven by considerations of who is 'the best person' to deliver it. This environment 'encourages specialization' (Theberge 2009b: 66). Conversely, at training camps athletes are likely to have access to a reduced support staff which, due to budgetary constraints, is most likely to be a single physiotherapist (despite recognition that the presence of a physician would be preferable/ideal). A central consequence is that the clinician has to be flexible in terms of duty – providing massage, acting 'up' in a physician role, but also undertaking menial duties (including driving, booking meals, moving equipment, etc.) reflecting a 'make-do' rather than 'optimal performance' philosophy and acting as a barrier to medical imperialism of the sports domain.

Within these structural restrictions to elite occupational healthcare, the interface with both coaches and athletes presents additional constraining factors. For instance, coaches play an important mediating role in both the delivery and uptake of healthcare provision. Gilmore and Sillince (2009) in their study of an English Football Premiership club, show how advances in sports medicine/sports science can be quickly disassembled due to managerial change. Similarly, Wagstaff et al. (2015) describe how the high turnover of personnel in elite sports teams make support staff vulnerable to externally imposed change. Moreover, (competitively successful) coaches rigidly stick to known routines and knowledge and fear disrupting programmes which they deem to currently be 'working' (Kerr 2012).

Elite athletes also exert significant influence over the medical provision they receive. Specifically, while Bundon and Clarke (2014: 133) note that there is 'an argument to be made that athletes could benefit from a more directed and strategic use of treatments', their primary critique is that 'elite athletes are operating in a system that pressures them to use everything at their disposal to optimise sport performance while simultaneously constraining their use through complex systems of delivery'. For example, elite athletes' use of CAMs is driven by what teammates are doing, prior socialization experiences (e.g. parents' use of these modalities) and concern that, 'by not trying a treatment an athlete might miss out' (Bundon and Clarke 2014: 128). Specifically, athlete demand strongly influences the provision and use of both massage and chiropractors. Athletes who define massage as 'absolutely essential and nonnegotiable' (Theberge 2012), come into conflict with (but ultimately defeat) administrators who are largely unconvinced of the evidence for its efficacy. Similarly, in debates about the contribution of chiropractors, 'concerns about the efficacy of spinal manipulation are resolved, not on the criterion of evidence-based medicine, but on the grounds of athletes' belief in its efficacy' (Theberge 2008: 31). Ultimately, administrators instruct medical staff to give athletes what they want, partly because preparation for competition is seen as holistic, and to go against the (relatively subjective) demands of the athlete would ultimately be counterproductive. The resultant occupational healthcare is 'a collage of coverage' (Bundon and Clarke 2014) which may entail specialists, may be highly individualized, but may not be expensive, sophisticated or innovative, and may have relatively limited evidence for its efficacy. A paradoxical inference of this is that, to some extent, the higher up the performance model of elite sport, and the greater the access to specialist/elite occupational healthcare, the more elements of 'irrational' provision persist.

None of this is to say that medicine is *never* rationally applied to sport, that elite occupational healthcare does not exist, or that commercial and international sport is not, particularly through aspects of experimentation, a 'field of medical mastery' (Young 1993: 376), but it does suggest that the most sophisticated forms of occupational medicine are certainly not the norm in sport, and are in fact something of a rarity. More accurately, we can say that provision is highly fragmented, of very variable quality and ultimately is frequently retarded more by the traditions and culture of sport than by limited financial resources. Problematizing Kotarba's thesis, the economic has invariably been subordinated to the cultural, and the rationalization of sports medicine has been socially contoured by 'subjective' positions that defy the 'objective' evidence. Although there is evidence that the medicalization of discourse has and is increasingly influencing the overall provision of sports medicine, the degree to which rationalization has impacted the specifics of medical provision in sport is rather more limited. Medicalization appears as likely to boost the position of para-medical professions and CAM providers as it is physicians themselves. In the next chapter we examine what this actually looks like in terms of medical practice, the degree to which medicine is relied upon to resolve the goals and issues of sports organizations.

Notes

1 According to Walk (2004) athletic trainers are equivalent to athletic therapists in Canada and sports physiotherapists in the UK. However, in contrast to sports physiotherapist (at least) he goes on to argue that a lot of athletic trainers' work is based on lay/sports knowledge and thus in contrast to the emphasis on evidence-based medicine that informs the physiotherapy discipline in general. See also Carter's (2009a) description of football trainers in England discussed later in this chapter.

2 FA regulations (2015) regarding CPD requirements are unclear and/or inconsistent. Regulation 2.5 states that in the Premier League 'each therapist' (it is not clear whether 'therapist' includes doctors as well as physiotherapists) must undertake a minimum of 36 hours CPD per year (18 hours of which must consist of formally approved courses), while in the Football League there are no CPD requirements listed for physiotherapists but a stipulation that team doctors fulfil a CPD programme 'as determined by the profession' (Regulation 3.4).

Chapter 8

The practice of 'elite' sports medicine

If the 'rational exploitation of science and medicine in the pursuit of competitive success' thesis is correct, one would expect this to be directly reflected in both the organizational commitment to medicine (and hence the *provision* of sports medicine), and the everyday utilization of biomedical actors in the resolution of the issues which those in the sporting world consider problematic (hence the *practice* of sports medicine). Yet, as outlined in Chapter 7, the majority of the provision of sports medicine is based on minimal economic investment, which results in a limited and low-skilled service. From this standpoint we continue a narrative of the medicalization of sport as relatively restricted, with sports medicine physicians far from central to the achievement of sports organizations' goals.

In contrast to what we now know of the provision of sports medicine, studies of the pain and injury experiences of athletes initially built on the view that performance was 'an important part of the *raison d'être*' of sports medicine (Waddington 1996: 185). For instance, in his pioneering work, Howard Nixon (1992: 128) contended that 'sportsnets' (the 'webs of interaction' that constitute the lived reality of sports clubs and include coaches, managers, medical staff, other athletes, spectators, administrators and investors) effectively conspired to coerce athletes to play through pain and with injury because competitive success is the priority of those most powerful in such figurations. But these studies also offered something of a paradox, for whilst sociologists have traditionally positioned medicine as a ubiquitous and imperialistic social institution (see Chapter 2), sports physicians often occupied relatively weak or subordinate roles and were relatively impotent actors within the broader power structure of sport. A picture emerged therefore of medical actors as neither very powerful nor autonomous in their practice. Indeed Walk argued that a central implication of Nixon's work on sportsnets, the culture of risk, etc., was that, 'medicine is practiced differently, more competently, and/or more ethically in nonsports contexts' (Walk 1997: 24). There are two broader sets of ideas that help us to understand this specific state of affairs: an Eliasian sociology of knowledge, and healthcare delivery trends indicative of a contemporary challenge to medical dominance.

Through historical comparison Elias demonstrates that 'only under specific societal conditions do people develop the capacity to manage their emotions in such a way, *in their relations with others*, as to make scientific detachment, which is a social accomplishment, possible' (Kilminster 2004: 27, original emphasis). More scientific forms of understanding always coexist and intermingle with more egocentric and emotionally-generated forms of knowledge, but generally the more pacified and predictable social life, the more rational and detached are the modes of thinking that predominate. Ultimately the ideas that become ascendant are the subject of social processes, surviving 'reality testing ... in the crucible of experience' (Elias, 1987: 56) rather than simply being externally and abstractly knowable. That which is 'known' is both rationally and socially constructed.

Illustrative of this broader perspective, and particularly pertinent for present purposes, is the distinction Elias (1974) makes between 'pure' and 'applied' science, and between the characteristics of the physical and social sciences. For Elias, the structural characteristics normally associated with medicine's social power more closely relate to pure as opposed to applied science. Pure biomedical science is associated with organizational coherence, specialist training, state licence and mandate, is frequently conducted in institutional settings that insulate the individual from outside interference (see for example the description of 'hospital medicine' in Chapter 2). 'Pure' biomedical science is thus relatively autonomous. Conversely, sports medicine, given the high dependence on a particular, non-clinical, 'patient group' (i.e. athletes), is fundamentally an applied science. Compounded by the absence of state support, which contributed to the fragmentation of sports medicine, this applied science is more likely to experience the intrusion of heteronomous perspectives; that is, be influenced by the 'values related to personal or social wishes and interests from outside the social institutions of science' (Mennell 1998: 166).

Moreover, part of what distinguishes the natural and social sciences, and what leads the former to dominate what Andrews (2008) calls the epistemological hierarchy, is the separation of subjects and objects of study. While in 'pure' natural science these aspects are distinctly and intentionally separated, in 'applied' natural science (and also social science) the objects are also the subjects; in other words, the investigators form part of the issues that they seek to resolve. It is essentially this to which Freidson (1970) refers in relation to the importance of the everyday work setting in shaping clinicians' actions (see Chapter 2). Specifically within the sport context, the key 'problem' (i.e. injury) is not defined solely in physiological, but in social, terms (i.e. production and performance). In many respects the injured athlete is deviant, but constraining the medicalization of this issue is the physical proximity of clinicians to the process of defining deviance.

As we will see in this and the following chapter, the medicalization of the treatment of sports injuries entails clashes between (crudely defined) scientific and lay bodies of knowledge. Stripped of the institutional buttresses that have characterized most of their professional lives, sports medicine clinicians are positioned as outsiders in this cultural milieu (relative to the coaches and athletes who might be defined as the established) and are vulnerable to the influence of their 'less scientific,' but more socially powerful, clients. Somewhat paradoxically, this leads both the provision and practice of healthcare in sport to become dominated by a profession (physiotherapy) which is markedly applied. Here, writ large, is the importance of social experience in the evaluation of competing bodies of knowledge.

Second, it should be noted that sports medicine as described in Chapter 7 exhibits a number of the characteristics that have been identified as posing fundamental challenges to medical dominance. In contrast to the 'golden age of doctoring' (McKinlay and Marceau 2002) sports medicine *qua* occupational medicine, exhibits considerable evidence of bureaucratic control over appointments, strong emphasis on the management as opposed to the treatment of conditions and, ultimately, a relatively weak market position. Also partly indicated already, but to be further elaborated in this and the subsequent chapter, are aspects of the managerial monitoring of medical practice and outcomes, the increasing influence of para-medical professions leading to jurisdictional contestation, the democratization of medical knowledge and patients' declining trust in medicine. This chapter illustrates both the strength of the challenge lay ideas and beliefs about sports injuries pose to medical scientific knowledge, and the dynamics of a 'new medical pluralism' (Cant and Sharma 1999). The latter is epitomized by the prevalence of MDTs in which healthcare providers, including practitioners of CAMs, are able to demonstrate more holistic and (in the eyes of patients) more efficacious interventions. Again, the sociology of knowledge is pertinent as rival professions mobilize competing narratives of their relative value. Importantly, however, we should not conceive of these characteristics as evidence of de-professionalization or proletarianization processes, for there is little evidence to suggest that sports medicine ever exerted the kind of social influence that originally inspired the medicalization thesis.

Building on these conceptual points, this chapter develops our understanding of the medicalization of sport by exploring the relative influence of medicine as *practised* within elite sport. It shows, through an examination of the dominant principles of sports medicine practice, how applied sports medicine is shaped by the 'heteronomous values' and ideologies that prevail in the sports subculture. It explores the enabling and constraining effects of the context of elite sport as a medical workplace, and the relationships practitioners have to negotiate with both their clients and co-workers. It concludes by focusing on the dynamics of the MDTs that predominate in sports medicine, assessing the relative influence of various medical providers, and ultimately arguing that the underpinning philosophies of physiotherapy practice relatively enable this profession to operate considerable jurisdictional leverage. What we see therefore are distinct limits to the scope of medicalization, particularly in relation to (sports) medicine's practice domain and actor identities.

The underpinning ideology of sports medicine practice

As noted in Chapter 1, the breadth and scope of the tasks and functions encompassed within contemporary sports medicine represent a considerable departure from the 'essential' defining goal of medicine; namely the relief of human suffering and the restoration of health (Edwards and McNamee 2006). Clinicians are aware of these contextual differences, if not before they enter this particular medical sphere, then immediately thereafter. As illustrated in the previous chapter, primary medical ethical principles such as confidentiality, privacy, patient autonomy and informed consent cannot be assumed to be operative in sports medicine (cf. Huizenga 1995; Waddington *et al.* 2001; Walk 1997). While existing studies show notable variations between some of the different contexts explored in Chapter 7 – college sport, commercial/professional sport and Olympic sports – the primary overarching issue is the conflicting ideological orientations of sport and medicine; the frequently contradictory goals of health and performance. As we see in this section, where these conflicting perspectives converge, they are invariably resolved in favour of the values traditional to sport rather than those espoused in medicine.

For example, at one end of the spectrum, research conducted in a 'large Canadian University', found that whilst major goal conflicts stemmed from clinician–athlete interactions, the practice conventions entailed clinicians operating a balance between the opposing cultures of risk and precaution (Safai 2003). Mediated by factors such as timing within the season, importance of upcoming events and the stage of an individual's varsity career, athletes tended to rely on lay knowledge as they engaged in self-diagnosis and self-prognosis. It was only after a process of intrapersonal negotiation, through which the costs and benefits of different courses of action were evaluated, that athletes would enter into the interpersonal negotiation of medical consultation. These negotiations entailed a relatively high degree of patient-centredness, with clinicians reporting: (a) the need to adapt sensitively their own position relative to the signs and signals omitted by the individual; and (b) recognition of the fundamental autonomy of the patient whom, both in theory and reality, they could ultimately only advise. Consequently, there was 'no evidence ... to suggest that sport medicine clinicians ... value the performance of the athlete above his/her health and wellbeing' (Safai 2003: 138), and thus 'the core process remains centred on the desire to heal' (Safai 2003: 143). In such cases the contextual demands impinge on the practice of sports medicine but do not fundamentally direct it.

However, more typically, Theberge's (2007) work with clinicians tasked with the healthcare of Canadian Olympic athletes concluded that performance was widely seen as the 'default position' with regard to the purpose of sports medicine. These clinicians similarly identified the relative autonomy of the athlete as central to shaping practice. Indicative of clinicians' inability to enforce patient compliance, they resorted to questioning the rationality of athletes' practice, characterizing this group as superstitious, corporeally vulnerable due to the stress under which their bodies are placed, and prone to making choices that reflect the desire to achieve psychological readiness rather than being informed by evidence-based principles of physiological efficacy. But, to an extent, the athletes are seen to 'get away' with these behaviours because clinicians come to learn that they principally evaluate health according to criteria defined by their athletic performance. In an important caveat to these findings, Theberge (2007) notes that a sense of the importance of health is rather more suppressed amongst physiotherapists, as evidenced in their failure to mention health at all until explicitly prompted, sometimes to the obvious embarrassment of the interviewee (this is explored in a later section of this chapter). With respect to the convergence of competing bodies of knowledge, it is clear that where doctors retain an emphasis on health relative to performance, they do so by re-conceptualizing the former to embrace lay evaluations of its contingency on the latter.

To date, the most striking examples of performance principles overriding health concerns occur in studies of commercial sport and English professional football in particular (Waddington 2000). Here, in contrast to Safai (2003) and Theberge's (2007) findings, the central negotiations over sports medicine practice were evident between coaches and clinicians. Examples included the instruction of clinicians to inconvenience players (e.g. by needlessly extending the time they are required to attend treatment) in order to 'incentivize' players to declare themselves fit to play, and diagnoses compromised by clinicians' awareness of sport-imposed (i.e. performance-based) time constraints. In more severe cases, coaches became directly involved in the management of injuries with either medical input circumvented through the coaching staff's control over logistics (e.g. arranging fitness tests so as to exclude the physiotherapist), or medical knowledge simply overridden by more powerful lay actors reliant upon experientially-derived knowledge. In a notable quote, in response to a question about the relative merits of the practice delivered in different working contexts, a football club physiotherapist stated, 'unequivocally, non-negotiable fact ... my private clients will get better quality treatment than the players' (cited in Waddington 2000: 66).

The degree to which medicine could be said to be practised differently in sports contexts was, and more broadly is, most evident in relation to the sanctity of the confidentiality of medical exchanges. Historically, the primacy of patient confidentiality has been central to medical ethics; it is the concluding item of the Hippocratic Oath. The importance of confidentiality stems from the notion that doctors should work wholly and exclusively on behalf of their patients and thus it is inextricably linked to patient autonomy. But confidentiality has been identified as one of the most important ethical issues in sports medicine (Stovitz and Satin 2006; Testoni *et al.* 2013), and empirically demonstrated to be amongst the ethical dilemmas most frequently encountered by sports doctors (Anderson and Gerrard 2005). For instance, a range of early studies, frequently based on personal recollections, identified the difficulties of directly transplanting medical ethical conventions into the sports domain (Dunn *et al.* 2007). Some suggested that problems could be resolved if one clearly distinguished between the roles of personal and team physician (Bernstein *et al.* 2004), or accepted the impossibility of preserving confidentiality in sports medicine, and thus explicitly made athletes aware of the inevitability that medical information would be shared with other medical, coaching and institutional personnel (Johnson 2004). Four contextual factors can be identified that encapsulate the social constraints on the operationalization of these ethical principles in sports medicine: clinicians' multiple and conflicting obligations; the openness of the physical environment in which sports medicine practice occurs; a policy context that routinely requires the public dissemination of otherwise privileged medical information; and a practice context that is multidisciplinary (embracing professionals with differing ethical norms), competitively-oriented and performance-driven (Malcolm 2016). Of eight existing studies of the management of confidentiality issues by sports clinicians (including doctors, physiotherapists and other paramedical professions) all include specific examples of practice contrary to the normal ethical principles of medicine, or an acceptance that in the context of sport individuals are forced to adapt such principles and thus fall below the standards of best practice (Malcolm 2016). Thus, the underpinning ideology of sports medicine practice conflicts with or problematizes the operationalization of the most fundamental aspects of the ethical basis of medical practice which, in turn, has traditionally been an important bolstering ideology for the social acceptance of medical power.

A striking element of this review of the underpinning ideologies of sports medicine practice is that where competing perspectives clash, there is actually little overt conflict. Clinicians in Olympic and professional sports medicine largely accommodate an ideology of performance that lies outside the traditional scope of medicine, and in so doing they either capitulate and abandon, or adapt and effectively circumvent, the spirit of medical ethical principles. There is no direct correlation between Kotarba's (2001) hierarchy of occupational medicine (elite, managed, primitive) and compliance with the traditional principles of medical practice and, indeed, across the threefold typology the actions of sports clinicians as providers of occupational medicine show a clear conflation of subjects and objects. Evidently, clinicians become embroiled in sporting issues, defining as well as legitimizing the 'deviant' injured athlete, and unable to stand apart from the consequences of their interventions and actions. The subsequent pressures force clinicians to modify their working practice in order to survive (a point which is further explored in relation to concussion in Chapter 9).

Elite sport as a medical workplace

Shaping the ideological principles that guide the practice of sports medicine are the distinct structural parameters of elite sport as a medical workplace. In this respect, Freidson's (1970) analysis of the medical profession is particularly apposite, especially his stress on the significance of 'everyday work settings' and, in particular, the degree to which doctors are amenable to lay or colleague control. However, we must also look, *pace* Abbott (1988), at the importance of inter-professional relations, for sports medicine's historical emphasis on multidisciplinarity provides distinct leverage. In sum, one can argue that context, clients and co-workers militate against the application of medical principles within the practice of sports medicine.

As described in Chapter 7, a common feature of the context in which many sports medicine clinicians in general, and doctors in particular, work is one of relative isolation from their professional colleagues (Malcolm 2006a, 2006b; Malcolm and Scott 2011; Waddington 2000). This lack of peer support is compounded by the necessity to conduct the majority of sports medicine practice in non-institutional settings that correlatively empower patients/managers. Specifically, in settings such as hospitals, the 'professional is on home territory whereas the patient is on "foreign" ground' (Freidson 1970: 225). By contrast, sports medicine is both metaphorically and literally practised 'in the field'.

Where that 'field' is commercially oriented, the pressures to generate income via a high media profile, 'may distort the focus of sport doctors such that they identify less with the health needs of the athlete and get pulled towards the aims of others involved in the sporting network' (Anderson and Jackson 2012: 246). In addition to studies that examined the coach and athlete as constraining forces on sports medical practice (see above), Anderson and Jackson identify sponsors and the media as factors that generate additional and competing obligations and serve to threaten the physicians' autonomy and thus professionalism. For instance, sports physicians speak about defacing sponsors' logos so that they can provide athletes with more suitable equipment, pressure from journalists to break patient confidentiality and the media-driven scheduling of sports events which may conflict with the health interests of participants. Sports medicine practice is therefore shaped by an awareness of the tripolar interdependence of the media, sponsors and athletes. Their mutual income generation revolves around the continued participation of the athlete, and is ultimately equally undermined by the athletes' withdrawal from the sport.

Implicit in this identification of converged interests, sports medicine is, to paraphrase Freidson (1970), a clients-dependent practice. Within sport, the physician is normally chosen on the basis of lay conceptions rather than medical-professional criteria of need and, tellingly in light of issues regarding confidentiality, Freidson (1970: 107) notes that in contexts such as these, 'professional standards are ... likely to be comparatively low'. As noted, studies have variously shown that coaches and athletes enter into relatively robust negotiations with clinicians, the former empowered by the convention of the 'coach as king' in professional team sport (Malcolm and Sheard 2002), and the latter by the dominance of a 'culture of risk' in which playing whilst injured is depicted as normal.

In this clients-dependent practice setting, we see a clash of lay and scientific bodies of knowledge. On the one hand, the medical scientific knowledge of the physician is relatively weakened by its applied rather than pure status whilst, on the other, lay knowledge of medical matters is empowered by the specificities of the practice context. Indeed sports clubs provide the kind of context in which Freidson (1970: 123–124) predicted that 'organized and persistent problems of patient management' are most likely to occur; namely, 'when patients are able to be in regular social interaction with each other, when they will all have the same general class of ailment about which they can exchange information, and when they share a relatively long-term, chronic prognosis'. Professionals in team sports are likely to experience the same *kinds* of injuries because they basically share the same working conditions, will have regular *interaction* with similar 'patients' (both because they share the same workplace where they train, travel and play as a team, and because they often see each other socially as well), and are injured so frequently that they share a relatively long-term *chronic prognosis*. In such contexts, therefore, lay knowledge becomes organized, systematic (Williams and Popay 1994) and relatively effectively mobilized. More egocentric, contextually esoteric, and immediacy-driven forms of knowledge (Elias 1987) predominate in this environment due to the relatively low levels of status and physical security (relatively short careers, frequency of injuries and player transfer, and the literal and public 'substitution' of individuals by those competing for a place in the team). Insecurity diminishes the ability of individuals to extract themselves from the potential threat that they face; what Elias (1987: 79) referred to as a 'double-bind' situation. The combined pressures from coaches and players lead doctors to recognize that their practice in the sports setting is, in many respects, different to that which they (aspire to) deliver in alternative working contexts.

Finally, sports medicine doctors find that their attempts to delineate their working practice are undermined by the presence of their co-health workers. As noted in Chapter 2, in order to protect its status as a self-directing and autonomous occupation, the medical profession has sought to direct and supervise the activities of related paramedical professions. However, as the discussion of provision showed (see Chapter 7), frequently this is not possible in sports medicine. Even where provision resembles elite occupational medicine, the paramedical professions of physiotherapy and sport/athletic therapy are likely to work a greater number of hours than their physician counterparts, and where the provision would better be described as 'managed' the therapist will often be able to demonstrate a higher level of sports-specific knowledge. Moreover, the means by which physicians conventionally control related occupations tends not to be available in sports medicine. Freidson (1970: 48–49) identifies four in particular:

- The technical knowledge of paramedical occupations is discovered, enlarged upon, or approved by doctors;
- The tasks performed assist rather than replace the focal tasks (i.e. those carried out by the doctor) of diagnosis and treatment;
- Paramedical workers are subordinate to, and organized/supervised by, doctors;
- The prestige assigned to paramedical workers is generally lower than that assigned to physicians.

All these conventional avenues of control may be subject to challenge in the domain of sports medicine.

As therapists provide the majority of healthcare in sports settings, they regularly work independently of doctors. This has been explicitly noted by both doctors and physiotherapists in a number of studies (Malcolm 2006a; Malcolm and Scott 2011; Theberge 2009a). Moreover, because of the differential time commitments of healthcare providers and the traditional reliance on certain treatment modalities, therapists have a high degree of control over doctors' access to the players and restrict doctors' ability to maintain open access to their clients. Specifically, it is usual only for the therapist to attend training and frequently also away fixtures, but even in competition where both healthcare providers are in attendance, it is the therapist who will usually be the first to enter the field of play to treat an injured player. Indeed, as Chapter 9 shows, exceptions to this frequently require explicit inter-professional negotiation. This is the consequence of therapists wielding – and being further enabled to wield – an unusually large influence over diagnosis, traditionally the foundation of medical jurisdictional claims (Jutel 2009). Additionally, while in the eyes of the public the physician is likely to be held in greater esteem, physicians are frequently demeaned by athletes (Malcolm and Sheard 2002; Walk 1997). Perhaps most importantly however, therapists are better aligned to what, in this context, becomes the 'focal task' for clinicians; namely performance.

The fundamental conservatism of medical practice – e.g. the ethical principle that one should 'first do no harm' (Devitt and McCarthy 2010) – restricts the degree to which the physician is predisposed to contribute to this inherently experimental realm. As we will see in the next section, this takes the primary orientation of practice out of the hands of medicine and locates it more centrally in the jurisdictional domain of the paramedical professions. Here, the practical advantages of being an essentially applied scientific profession become evident.

The dynamics of multidisciplinary healthcare teams in sport

As we saw in the conclusion to Chapter 7, where resources permit, the primacy attached to athletes' healthcare preferences can lead to a proliferation in the provision of treatment modalities. Even where this is not evident, it remains common (as suggested above) for two or more healthcare providers (e.g. a doctor and physiotherapist) to work alongside each other. To some extent this is characteristic of wider developments in healthcare practice, where economic arguments have been mobilized to justify an expanded division of labour which, in turn, evokes a fundamental challenge to the traditional dominance of the medical profession. Recent developments in physiotherapy exemplify this. Initially, medical policing of physiotherapy's administration and accreditation, and through the categorization of massage as akin to a prescription drug, physiotherapists were effectively 'forced to depend on them [doctors] for work' (Larkin 1983: 119; see also Nicholls and Cheek 2006). New funding models, health care policies, advocacy of key groups and support from the medical profession have changed that and had a direct impact on working practices (Bury and Stokes 2013). Sports physiotherapy has been described as particularly well placed to respond to future healthcare needs due to the increasing state emphasis on promoting health through physical activity (CSP 2008), and has been identified as a field of considerable growth and 'a particularly lucrative area of specialisation' (APA 2011). Recent manifestations of this include the ability for physiotherapists to act as 'first practitioners' so that patients/clients may seek services 'without referral from another healthcare professional' (Bury and Stokes 2013: 450).

Contrary to the logic of professional boundary contestation, the emphasis in MDTs on sharing knowledge and responsibility and actively fostering cooperation and collaboration (Reid *et al.* 2004; Suddick and De Souza 2006), means that relations are frequently relatively harmonious. For instance, a study of nursing–medical staff relations attributed interprofessional cooperation to the 'organisational turbulence' of hospital work (Allen 1997: 506). In the relatively insulated working environment of intensive care, spatial separation fosters cross-professional identity as 'an occupational division of labour is rhetorically and practically obscured, while an organisational division is rhetorically and practically reinforced' (Carmel 2006: 155). The lived experiences of professional boundary work are often less conflict-ridden than assumed (Nancarrow and Borthwick 2005).

This is nowhere more evident than in the practice of sports medicine. For instance, inter-professional relations have been described as 'collegial and smooth' (Theberge 2008: 24) due to the shared athlete-centric model of work in Canadian elite sports medicine provision (see Malcolm and Scott 2011 for a comparative analysis of British elite sports medicine). Part of that, undoubtedly, is due to recognition of the legitimate and acceptable limits of such a challenge. Sports physiotherapists have referred to doctors' central role in the administration of drugs (i.e. writing prescriptions and giving injections; cf. Cooper et al. 2011), deployment of technology (particularly, MRI scans) and their ultimate authority to make 'final' diagnoses. In so doing they express a clear 'desire to have their boundary incursions legitimated by doctors' (Malcolm and Scott 2011: 519). However, it would also be true to say that the pressures of the sports working context have been found to drive healthcare professionals together as they forge alliances for mutual support in opposition to non-healthcare members of the sportsnet (Malcolm and Sheard 2002; Waddington 2000).

Where MDTs incorporate a broader group of professions, and where the professional hierarchy is less well historically established, competition typically becomes manifest in the legitimation discourses/jurisdictional narratives professions use to distinguish themselves from others. Sanders and Harrison (2008) found that those who treated patients with heart failure emphasized six main narrative themes: reference to the scientific basis of work; identification of particular skills and expertise; the holistic and patient-centred nature of practice; the provision of care and emotional support; organizational efficiency and accountability; and claims to competence. Similarly, sports physiotherapists practising with British Olympic athletes were found to mobilize notions of holism to contrast their own efficacy with that of the perceived limitations of doctors (Malcolm and Scott 2011). In physiotherapists' claims to such things as competence, organizational efficiency and patient-centred care, these findings replicate the 'fairly clear inverse relationship' identified between 'occupations' respective location in the professional status hierarchy and the number and variety of legitimating discourses employed' (Sanders and Harrison 2008: 304).

However, such debates are perhaps even more pronounced where considerable overlap exists between the claimed scope of practice of the various therapists who provide MSK treatment. In recognition of the absence of clear boundaries, Canadian physiotherapists, athletic therapists and chiropractors engaged in extended jurisdictional boundary work through rhetorical strategies identifying their relative breadth of practice, the legitimacy of their qualifications and their sports-specific specialism (Theberge 2009a). Given their closeness, each could argue for the redundancy of the others. Consequently, claims to distinct forms of legitimacy were important. Each profession was, ultimately, distinguished on the basis of its historical relationship with: (a) sport; and (b) medicine. Ultimately, it was physiotherapy's claim to the latter which in particular enabled it to become viewed as the dominant profession.

But as Elias (1987) suggests, just as such knowledge claims cannot be evaluated solely in relation to a priori criteria such as 'truth', nor are they simply a form of abstract discourse. Rather knowledge is ultimately judged on social criteria and in particular on the basis of what humans find 'consistently works' (Mennell 1998: 161) as they go about their everyday lives. Knowledge only survives if humans believe that it has specific use-value. This is where physiotherapy is advantaged relative to medicine in sport, where the use value of the latter may be longer term and therefore less immediately apparent. Congruence between the traditional practice philosophy of physiotherapy and the raison d'être of sports cultures is fundamentally what enables this profession to exert a level of influence that defies the traditional hierarchy of medicine and its allied professions. In particular, it is claimed that physiotherapy practice is strongly influenced by experiential learning (compared, for example, to medicine where innovations are largely laboratory-led), and that interactions tend to be highly collaborative, educative and foster mutuality (Jensen et al. 2000; Parry 2009). In focusing on functionality of the patient's body, physiotherapy incorporates patients' embodied experiences more than conventional medical examination does (Thornquist 1995), and consequently expertise is judged according the 'reasoning strategies that could be used to solve problems' (Jensen et al. 2000: 30).

Specifically, physiotherapists contrast their immersion into their sport-related practice with that experienced in, for example, public health care settings (Scott and Malcolm 2015). In the former, their involvement appears in every facet of the treatment process (injury prevention, rehabilitation and performance enhancement), and results in the prolonged engagement with 'patients' who are never discharged. Thus, a physiotherapist's typical treatment scenario has been described as follows:

> What you might do is get someone in the first or second stage [of injury] and work with a coach in the third stage. You could have them for the first stage and then hand them on to strength and conditioning in the second stage and then pick them back up in the final stage.... Then you're involved in the injuries, rehabilitation, injury prevention and then out in the field when they are competing.
>
> (Quoted in Scott and Malcolm 2015: 552)

Through this elision of treatment and training, sports physiotherapists are able to continually and organically expand their knowledge and become closely aligned to the performance goals of the broader figuration. They solely work towards and are seen to contribute to the resolution of 'problems' identified by athletes and coaches. Often a strong rapport develops between patient and physiotherapist, as does a degree of emotional reliance, as evident for example in athletes' requests for the clinician to accompany them in consultations with physicians. The closeness of these relationships insulates the physiotherapist from the broader critiques of the lack of efficacy of modern biomedicine and ultimately protects them from the fundamental problem of treatment failure. As one sports physiotherapist described:

> I have said things to athletes that I probably shouldn't have said and I have made diagnoses that were wrong. I have bet my reputation that there was nothing wrong with an athlete's knee and he ended up having an ACL rupture!... Ultimately, if an athlete keeps their faith in you and ... they still come back to you, then it means you are doing something. Because if you weren't good at those other things they would walk away because clinically you have made the biggest mistake and the biggest call of your life. But for some reason they come back. Why? That's the other bits. You can't always quantify it.
>
> (Quoted in Scott and Malcolm 2015: 554)

Thus,

> close physical contact and experiential learning foster physiotherapist-patient mutuality, locates the physiotherapist as integral to rehabilitation, and therefore physiotherapy as inherent to performance and enhancement ... [which in turn] leads to trusting and collaborative healthcare relations ... and enables sports physiotherapists to be seen to be equipped to solve patients' problems.
>
> (Scott and Malcolm 2015: 551)

Conclusion

While in Chapter 7 we saw how the provision of sports medicine is highly fragmented, of varying quality, and frequently retarded by the traditions and culture of sport as much as limited financial resources, here we have shown that the practice of sports medicine is similarly shaped by the heteronomous values of the world of sport (i.e. performance) as opposed to traditional medical principles (i.e. the promotion of health). The influence of medicine is fundamentally curtailed by the context, clients and co-workers with which sports medicine physicians are necessarily interdependent. In particular, the latter (most notably physiotherapists) are empowered by practice traditions which emphasize experiential learning for patient-driven problem resolution while physicians are in some respects constrained by the primacy of educational qualifications, claims to esoteric expert status, and the relatively autonomous evaluation of the 'importance' or severity of conditions. Sports medicine physicians experience many of the society-wide challenges to medical dominance, but with little of the institutional legitimation or support enjoyed by their non-sport counterparts. Ironically, the close association of medicine with 'pure' science is a relative hindrance in comparison with the fundamentally applied, literally 'hands on' (Barclay 1994) character of physiotherapy, which is more highly valued in 'crucible of [sporting] experience' (Elias 1987: 56).

Of course, that physicians are commonly to be found in these everyday work settings is a consequence of the ubiquity of medicalization as discourse. Indeed, again ironically, the fact that physiotherapists can draw on a historical association with medicine to assert dominance in contexts where competing MSK (musculoskeletal) therapists populate MDTs is testament to the society-wide influence of this broader narrative which, in turn, has played a major part in structuring these para-medical professions. But what the examination of the practice of sports medicine fundamentally reveals is the disjuncture between the prevalence of this ideology and the application of medical techniques and the mobilization of medical actors in the routine delivery of sports medicine. We develop this analysis in Chapters 9 and 10, where we explore the dynamics of two more tightly delineated examples of sports medicine practice which, on the face of it, more closely rely on the expertise of the medical profession: namely the management of concussion and the implementation of cardiac screening.

Chapter 9

The medicalization of concussion

Concussion is the term used historically to describe relatively low force impacts that cause the brain to shake or rotate within the skull. As such, concussion is a form of mild Traumatic Brain Injury (mTBI). Typically, concussions result in 'rapid onset of short-lived impairment of neurological function that resolves spontaneously' (McCrory *et al.* 2013: 250) although some cases may evolve over days and there is no standard timeline for resolution. The primary symptoms are functional and include headache, disorientation and instability, cognitive impairment (slurred speech, memory loss, slowed reactions), sleep disturbance and loss of consciousness. If concussion does entail underlying structural injury to the brain, medical technology (e.g. neuroimaging) is not sufficiently developed at this time to consistently enable its detection (McCrory *et al.* 2013). The 'vague and heterogeneous symptoms' (McNamee *et al.* 2015: 193) make both diagnosis and prognosis complicated and contested. While debates over mTBIs have impacted on boxing's specific interdependence with medicine for over 100 years (see Chapter 3), heightened concern about concussion across a wide range of contact team sports has been one of the most visible manifestations of the medicalization of sport in the twenty-first century; and the subject of a 2015 Hollywood film starring Will Smith which grossed in excess of $44 million.

Concussion, moreover, provides a particularly revealing illustration of the complexities of the medicalization of sport. On the one hand we see elements of medical imperialism as the sports medicine community has acted effectively not only to define concussion as an issue in need of addressing, but as an issue which does and should fall under the provenance of medicine. As we will see, at the conceptual level the medical paradigm has been particularly successful in structuring public and media understanding of concussion. Correlatively, aspects of elite sport that conflict with the sport–health ideology, and in particular cultures of risk, have been opened up to public scrutiny. Medicalization has also been evident at the institutional level as biomedical procedures are increasingly used to administer the social problem of concussion in sport. In this respect, medicine has been successful in invoking regulatory and organizational responses from sports governing bodies. However, the expansion of jurisdictional influence at the interactional level has been less successful due to the inability of medicine to live up to the professional promise of authoritative and definitive knowledge. Indeed, on a microsocial level, the individual biomedical actors may experience 'deprofessionalization' as a consequence of engagement with concussion issues. While Chapters 7 and 8 explored constraints in the scope and status of medicine due to the clash of medical knowledge with that of employers, patients and para-medical co-workers, this chapter highlights how such interdependencies impact on sports medicine through the reshaping of (medical) knowledge and thus practice. Consequently, we explore how concussion discourse has become increasingly medicalized, how this has impacted upon sports governing bodies and the media, and finally on those charged with implementing concussion treatment protocols in sport.

The medicalization of concussion discourse

Concern about concussion within the sports medicine community became increasingly prominent from the late 1990s. A central figure in this broader movement was the Australian neurologist and sports physician, Paul McCrory. A club doctor in the Australian Football League (AFL), and consultant to a range of sports organizations, McCrory was editor of the BJSM from 2001–2008 and used this position to centre sports medicine in the public understanding and clinical management of concussion injuries. He criticized existing research on concussion for being 'anecdotal ... bizarre rather than reflecting established medical principles' and argued that the field was plagued by a 'neuromythology' derived from folk wisdom, methodologically flawed medical research, and media exposés of athletes' experiences of head trauma (McCrory 2001a: 82). The field, he argued, was hampered by the lack of any 'existing animal or other experimental model that accurately reflects a sporting concussive injury' (McCrory et al. 2005: 197). Knowledge, rather, was based upon research on head injuries sustained in boxing and motor vehicle accidents, which was misleading because: (a) the frequency of repetitive head trauma in boxing is thought to pose 'unique risks'; and (b) collisions in sports such as rugby union involve much lower acceleration–deceleration forces than do motor vehicle accidents. McCrory further made the case that a proliferation of scales designed to assess the severity of head injuries (there were over 20 in 2000) meant that clinicians and athletes were often confused by conflicting advice (McCrory 1999). It was, for instance, unclear whether concussion injuries should be graded according to the presence/absence of particular symptoms (with loss of consciousness traditionally defined as the most severe) rather than their duration (McCrory *et al.* 2005). While it was argued that there was no conclusive evidence that sustaining several concussions over a sporting career necessarily resulted in permanent damage (McCrory 2001a), medical and lay concerns largely stemmed from fears over so-called 'second impact syndrome' (where subsequent head injuries become increasingly regular and/or severe) and the 'unstated fear' that athletes who are repeatedly concussed will ultimately experience cognitive decline similar to that of the 'punch drunk' boxer (McCrory 2001b: 380).

Through these critiques, McCrory became central to a process whereby medical knowledge of concussion would become more unified and thus coherent and increasingly seen as distinctive and distinguished, while the influence of 'folk wisdom' or lay knowledge would concomitantly be reduced. The single most tangible outcome of McCrory's actions was the establishment in 2001 of a series of international conferences on sports concussion that have produced a succession of Agreement/Consensus Statements on Concussion in Sport. McCrory has been the lead author for all but the first of these statements. The fifth and latest of these conferences is planned for October 2016. These 'concussion consensus statements ... serve as an important part of sports medicine's increasing professionalization' (McNamee *et al.* 2015: 200).

Although it is recognized that knowledge limitations remain (which, as we will see, have significant practical ramifications), the last decade has witnessed important biomedical developments in the understanding of concussion in sport. Fundamental to this has been a process akin to what Armstrong (1995) describes as surveillance medicine, as a range of epidemiological surveys have seen the condition transform from 'the hidden epidemic' (Marshall and Spencer 2001) to the recognition that in some sports it is the most frequently recorded injury-type (Kirkwood *et al.* 2015). Incidence varies considerably across surveys, but concussion is undoubtedly most prevalent in high-speed contact sports such as the various football codes (American football, Australian Rules football, association football, rugby union and rugby league) and ice hockey (Fuller *et al.* 2014). The findings of individual studies make stark reading. Delaney *et al.* (2008) and Fraas *et al.* (2013) found that nearly half of footballers and rugby (union) players experienced at least one concussion per year, while Partridge (2014) cites Australian studies which indicate that AFL and National Rugby League (NRL) teams are likely to experience between five and seven concussions per season. Price *et al.* (2012) anticipate that a professional football squad will experience one concussion approximately every month and Broglio *et al.* (2010) extrapolated from their study of Italian footballers to estimate that there are 2.1 million soccer-related concussions worldwide each year. However, the incidence of concussion in American football is thought to be almost double that of any other sport, with official

National Football League (NFL) statistics recording a concussion once every 2.5 games (Casson *et al.* 2010). It has been estimated that there could be as many as four million concussion injuries per year in the US alone (McGannon *et al.* 2013).

The concerns over concussion that heighten its impact as a social issue are fuelled by three key factors. First, many athletes experience repeat concussions during the season (Delaney *et al.* 2008). Second, it is widely recognized that epidemiological research fails to fully capture the frequency of concussion. Studies in English professional rugby union (Malcolm 2009), US high school sport and Canadian youth ice hockey (cited in McNamee *et al.* 2016) indicate that participants frequently under-present their symptoms. The reasons identified for this – namely: (a) perceptions that their condition is not serious enough; (b) reluctance to leave the game and/or let down teammates; or (c) disbelief that a concussion has occurred (Broglio *et al.* 2010; Fraas *et al.* 2013; McCrea *et al.* 2004) – all pathologize the athlete and leave the broader structure of sport and (in)action of clinicians unchallenged. Third, the incidence of concussion amongst youth players appears to be similar to that in elite sport (Kirkwood *et al.* 2015). Indeed, the heightened concern over youth concussion has led to the development of separate assessment tools for under-12s, and the recommendation of more cautious management protocols. Children who return to play (RTP) on the day of injury are thought to suffer more marked cognitive deterioration (Makdissi *et al.* 2014) and thus it is believed that children may require a longer recovery period than adults (McCrory *et al.* 2013). While empirical evidence to support the more conservative management of youth concussions is often lacking (McNamee *et al.* 2015), it was specifically the concern over concussion in this population that attracted Barack Obama's attention to this issue (see Chapter 1). Concussion, therefore, is increasingly seen to threaten the integrity of the sport–health ideology.

However, this growing concern is (partly) an inevitable consequence of the impact of biomedical investigation. Epidemiological research does not simply reflect incidence, but fundamentally changes human understanding of the condition and contributes to its construction as a social issue (Petersen and Lupton 1996). Indicatively, there is growing concern that the repercussions of concussive injuries are wider-ranging and more enduring than previously believed. The term 'chronic postconcussion syndrome' has been introduced to describe symptoms so persistent that an athlete is forced to retire from sport (Jordan 2013: 228). As awareness grew, so increasing numbers of athletes and their families began to speculate that the mental health of some retired players (manifest in depression, irritability, mood volatility, etc.) was attributable to the impact of career-long concussions. In some cases concussion has been implicated in sport-related suicides (Malcolm and Scott 2014), and athletes and their families have requested post-mortem brain analyses. Some of these, such as the case of

Dave Duerson, an ex-NFL player who shortly before shooting himself sent a text to his family requesting that they submit his body for neuropathological investigation, have found evidence of chronic traumatic encephalopathy (CTE), 'a degenerative brain disease linked to repeated head trauma and characterised by dementia-like symptoms, memory disturbances, and speech problems' (Partridge 2014: 66). In Britain, the *Jeff Astle Foundation* was formed following a coroner's ruling that the former professional footballer's death (aged 59), (probably) stemmed from his repeated heading of the ball (Britten 2002). In 2013 the NFL 'tentatively agreed' a $765 million settlement with over 4500 former players who had accused the league of both mismanaging players' neurological health and concealing evidence of the long-term risks (Associated Press 2013). Evidence suggests that former NFL players are three times more likely than the general population to suffer a neurodegenerative disease (Partridge and Hall 2014: 2)

The medicalization of concussion has both been consolidated by, and extends to, the incorporation of the para-medical healthcare groups into the generation and analysis of knowledge. Sports psychology has focused on 'the emotional trauma ... pain and anxiety' following mTBI (McGannon *et al.* 2013: 891). For instance, a study of five National Hockey League (NHL) players who retired due to head injuries demonstrated 'the long-term effects of concussions on multiple quality of life domains', as respondents experienced debilitating physical symptoms for up to 14 years and psychological impacts such as anxiety, depression, social withdrawal, loss of identity and suicidal ideation (Caron *et al.* 2013: 176). While psychologists are critical of the dominance of 'using quantitative methodologies to describe the physiological and neurocognitive outcomes' (Caron *et al.* 2013: 169), and note that the dominance of neurologists in the monitoring of concussed athletes contradicts recommendations to treat concussion across its psychological, social and cultural as well as physical dimensions (McGannon *et al.* 2013), their concerns underscore the jurisdictional hegemony of medicine in this domain. For instance, while player narratives contain criticisms of individual medical personnel, the fact that physician intervention was crucial to the retirement of all of Caron *et al.*'s (2013) interviewees illustrates how biomedicine is accepted as the disciplinary lead. At the conceptual level, 'folk wisdom' (McCrory 2001a) of concussion has been discredited.

The medicalization of concussion practice

Shifts in biomedical understanding have led to changes in the regulation of concussion in various sports. Historically the International Rugby Board (IRB) has been seen as leading the way in the precautionary regulation of concussion. At the beginning of the twenty-first century, the IRB adopted a definition of concussion that both operated conservatively and resonated with lay knowledge. Specifically, the IRB did not differentiate between severity grades but recommended, for instance, that 'being unaware of what happened, even for a few moments at the time of the injury is the most consistent sign that the player is or has been concussed'. Any rugby player suspected of sustaining a concussion was prohibited from playing and training for a minimum of three weeks and was only allowed to resume 'when symptom free and declared fit after a proper medical examination' (IRB 2008: regulation 10.1.1).

Development of international consensus statements and Concussion in Sport Guidelines (CISG) led to a degree of regulatory convergence across sports. The CISG standardized the definition of concussion such that a direct blow to the head and loss of consciousness (LOC) were ruled out as diagnostic prerequisites (indeed it is now argued (e.g. Casson 2010) that approximately only 10% of concussions entail LOC). A 'gold standard' management protocol has been produced that recommends that athletes undergo baseline cognitive and concussion symptom testing; be assessed using a standardized Sports Concussion Assessment Tool (SCAT); and be wholly asymptomatic throughout a six-phase graduated RTP programme, lasting a minimum of six days and overseen by a medical practitioner.

The degree to which these recommendations have been adopted varies but most contact team sports have been affected. In 2011, Australia's AFL and NRL implemented concussion management systems based on the CISG. To encourage conservative management, rugby league teams are awarded an additional substitution when a player is withdrawn exhibiting concussion symptoms. The response of the IRB has been somewhat contradictory, not participating in the initial international conference, and subsequently supplementing the gold standard management protocol with the more contentious 'head injury bin', which permits temporary substitutions to facilitate the diagnosis of concussion. Initial criticism of this policy development was led by the IRB's own former medical advisor, Barry O'Driscoll, who resigned over the issue arguing that the head injury bin would lead to greater flexibility and inevitably therefore less conservative injury management.[1]

In football, and despite FIFA backing for the consensus statements (one of three original partners with the International Ice Hockey Federation (IIHF) and IOC), the English FA were slow to adopt the CISG. The 2010–2011 and 2011–2012 medical regulations effectively enabled concussed players to RTP within a few minutes. Given the relatively low level of sport-specialist knowledge amongst football club medical personnel (see Chapter 7), it was perhaps not surprising that 55.6% of football clubs did not routinely follow the recommended CISG, that 'Only 21% of teams routinely record an approved preseason cognitive score ... only 42% complete the appropriate postconcussion assessment', and indeed that a quarter of club doctors had no knowledge of the operant consensus statement

(Price *et al.* 2012: 1). The 2012–2013 regulations did adopt the SCAT and a six-phase graduated RTP (though not time-limited), recommended the use of baseline testing, but deferred autonomy to clinical judgement and individualized treatment to allow an almost immediate RTP if symptoms rapidly resolved. Following a number of high profile incidents (e.g. when Tottenham goalkeeper Hugo Lloris continued in a game having clearly been knocked unconscious), regulations were revised to mirror the gold standard protocol noted above. The guidelines on the management of concussion and head injuries cover 13 of the 16 pages of the FA's (2015) medical regulations. The phased adoption of the CISG suggests that public relations have been rather more significant in driving change than the advancement of biomedical knowledge.

Perhaps the most radical changes however have occurred in American football. A 2005 NFL-commissioned study declared the league's existing protocol – following the American Academy of Neurology's 1997 concussion guidelines, players could RTP if symptoms had resolved within 15 minutes – too *conservative* (McNamee and Partridge 2013). Due to legal challenges the NFL subsequently moved more into line with the rest of the sporting world with baseline cognitive testing and the prohibition of any player diagnosed as concussed (assessed relative to the baseline testing) from re-entering the field of play. Additionally, an independent athletic trainer helps identify suspected concussions from the stand, and an NFL-appointed neurological specialist is pitch-side to aid team physicians' diagnoses (NFL Head, Neck and Spine Committee and Bradley 2013). Players then pass through a five-stage graduated RTP programme, although critics note that there are no time limits on how quickly the phases can be completed. Finally, players are required to obtain clearance from a non-NFL employed physician prior to re-selection. The NFL's concussion protocol was compiled in consultation with the NFL Players Association, NFL Physicians Society and the Professional Football Athletic Trainers Society (Clarke 2015) but not, it should be noted, the ACSM. Again, change has largely been driven by factors external to advances in biomedical knowledge.

Many sports have also changed their rules of play to reduce the incidence of head injury. Rugby union has increasingly restricted the height of tackling and sought to reduce contact between airborne players, particularly where this may lead a player to fall head first to the ground. In ice-hockey, the IIHF has restricted tackling that includes body contact from particular directions (e.g. behind) and/or that is targeted at the head (McGannon *et al.* 2013). Casson *et al.* (2010) list 11 changes to NFL regulations between 1995 and 2009, restricting specific tactics, player formations and forms of contact. Association football and lacrosse have been more reluctant to invoke rule changes. FIFA's rules have not fundamentally changed, although in 2015 the US governing body prohibited under-10s from heading the ball (de Menezes 2015). Lacrosse authorities have been criticized for the inequity of having compulsory hard helmets for males but not for females (Schwarz 2011). It should be noted however that the international consensus on, and evidence for the efficacy of, the introduction of new forms of equipment (e.g. helmets, padding, etc.) is ambiguous. So-called 'risk compensation theory' is the underpinning rationale for this; namely the idea that the better protected an individual feels, the more carefree/reckless they may play, leading to increased injury incidence (Malcolm *et al.* 2004). NFL players are both the most heavily protected and frequently concussed athletes.

The changing CISG, the more extensive adoption of standardized concussion management practices and shifts in the rules of play, suggest that the medicalization of concussion discourse has been fundamental to the increasing regulation of player health. However, the reluctance of sports administrators to alter rules has been a notable element of resistance to the changing biomedical knowledge and regulatory recommendations. Indeed, indicative of the delicate balance of power, the latest consensus document encourages rule changes to enhance player safety, with the proviso that medical assessment should avoid, 'affecting the flow of the game or unduly penalizing the player's team' (McCrory *et al.* 2013: 6). We will explore the actual impact of such changes on the everyday work settings of sports medicine clinicians and their athlete-patients shortly, but first we look at the media's engagement with concussion which, in almost all respects, has essentially fuelled the medicalization process.

Concussion and the media

Public responses to the medically inspired, concussion-related, rule changes in sport have been largely supportive of biomedical intervention. This is evident in some of the more notable media reports in recent years. These include the post-retirement revelations of rugby players Shontayne Hape (Deane 2014) and Rory Lamont (Ferguson 2013), and the head injuries sustained by Aaron Rodgers of the Green Bay Packers in the NFL (Anderson and Kian 2012) and Sidney Crosby of the Pittsburgh Penguins in the NHL (McGannon *et al.* 2013). Despite some transatlantic differences, media coverage provides a coherent overarching narrative, i.e. that sport practice is problematic and the solution to the social issue of concussion in sport is increased or improved medical surveillance. To paraphrase McNamee *et al.* (2015: 191) it appears that lay confidence in sports medicine and science over this issue tends to be 'uncritical and naïve'. Four specific themes in the press coverage converge towards this conclusion.

Concussion remains a considerable concern

It was reported that Hape, who played international rugby league and union for New Zealand and England respectively, was forced to retire from sport due to 'constant migraines, sensitivity to light and sound, irritability, memory loss and depression' (Deane 2014). He claimed to have suffered approximately 20 concussions during his career before incurring three head injuries in quick succession which meant that, 'dosing up on smelling salts, Panadol, high caffeine sports drinks and any medical drugs like that to try to stop the [symptoms] … was the only way I could get through training and matches'. Similarly, press coverage of Rodgers' essentially unilateral decision to remove himself from an NFL game demonstrates the emergence of more conservative attitudes towards concussion (Anderson and Kian 2012), while Crosby's coverage represented a 'cautionary tale' in problematizing the culture of sport which led to his RTP despite manifest symptoms of concussion in consecutive matches (McGannon *et al.* 2013: 895).

Regulation is too weak and/or can be circumvented

Crosby's concussion became an explicitly political platform, invoking a broader debate about whether (recent) regulatory changes in the NHL were sufficient to safeguard players. Hape and Lamont both stated that it was widely known that players manipulated rugby union's pre-season baseline cognitive testing to give themselves a greater chance of subsequently avoiding a diagnosis of concussion and/or appearing asymptomatic more quickly. Lamont (cited Ferguson 2013) argued that cognitive testing was therefore counter-productive in that negative tests provided only false reassurance of health.

Players are largely seen as responsible for regulation failure

While Hape and Lamont both provided accounts of significant pressure from coaching staff during their careers including, in Hape's case, attempts to overrule medical advice and return the player after a brief rest period, in both cases the press primarily focused on the aforementioned revelation of players' rigging of test results. Similarly, the coverage of Rodgers' case suggested that players were the main resistance to change, epitomized in one players' testimony that 'that's how we are' (cited in Anderson and Kian 2012: 163). The mismanagement of Crosby was attributed to widespread misunderstanding of the dangers but, notably, there was no suggestion that the player had been pressured by coaches or medical staff.

Concussion remains a condition shrouded in uncertainty

The press frequently described concussion as a unique injury due to its (frequent) invisibility and unpredictability. Media coverage of the Rodgers' case focused on the contested nature of the assessment of the health risks related to concussion. Similarly, the Pittsburgh Penguins' manager attempted to stave off criticism of the club's handling of Crosby's injury by emphasizing the complexity of the condition and the need 'to learn more' (McGannon *et al.* 2013: 897). In Hape's case, the media focused on the inability to contain, control or resolve symptoms.

These four themes converge to enhance the role of medicine in the resolution of public concerns over sporting concussions. While attention to the frequency and severity of injuries fundamentally problematizes the sport–health ideology, emphasis on the culture of risk in sport and the responsibility of athletes and administrators for the current failure of concussion regulation seems to militate against a more significant questioning of existing practice. Where clinicians are criticized (e.g. in the case of Crosby) individual actors rather than the profession per se are the target. Sports medicine is represented as the unequivocal guardian of a sport–health ideology threatened by the practices of sports subculture. Ironically perhaps, the perceived uncertainty over concussion does not undermine faith in the efficacy of medicine but justifies its expanded jurisdiction. For instance, the media express faith in the deployment of neurologists and are generally keen to report on innovative technology, such as wearable impact-measuring equipment and a 'breathalyzer' test to detect concussion (BBC 2015b; Webb 2014). These narratives are ultimately intertwined with the potential of biomedicine to resolve how these 'deviant' (i.e. injured) athletes should be treated.

However, as discussed in the next section, uncertainty fundamentally restricts the degree to which clinicians can effectively manage head injuries and therefore medicalize concussion-related practice. Moreover, contrary to press accounts, uncertainty is neither temporary nor ephemeral but inherent to the discipline and profession of medicine. Consequently, medical actors may be constrained by the broader working context, particularly when the contradictions between medicine's discursive claims and the lived experience of efficacy are exposed. In the next section we look at the biomedical actors tasked with the responsibility for implementing concussion regulations in a practice context which, we have seen (Chapter 8), exhibits significant barriers to the influence of medical knowledge.

Medicalization, concussion and healthcare providers

Although concussion in sport has been relatively effectively medicalized at both the conceptual level and in the institutional administration of concussion as a social/sporting issue, its micro-level management remains more problematic. Press coverage of concussion cases provides some evidence of this, with clinicians criticized for their (in)decisions (e.g. in the Rodgers' and Lloris cases). Yet while press narratives publicly recognize the degree of uncertainty over concussion, they fail to reflect its impact on those tasked with the clinical management of concussion. Uncertainty fundamentally undermines the professional project of medicine, hampering clinicians' attempts to operationalize concussion guidelines in their everyday practice settings in sport. Evidence for the medicalization of concussion at this level is considerably weaker and indeed elements of de-professionalization if not anti-medicalization exist. The notion of uncertainty resonates with Elias's sociology of knowledge discussed in Chapter 8, illustrating the interdependence of more scientific and emotionally-generated forms of knowledge, and the relative power of established and outsider groups (Elias and Scotson 1994) in socially determining what constitutes 'truth'.

Contrary to the medical profession's claims to authoritative knowledge, 'uncertainty is inherent in medicine' (Fox 2000: 409). Uncertainty is a normal feature of becoming and being a medical practitioner. Medical students experience uncertainty stemming from the limitations of medical knowledge (*epistemological uncertainty*), uncertainty stemming from the awareness of being unable to master all aspects of medical knowledge and practice (*clinical uncertainty*), and uncertainty stemming from the inability to distinguish between the two. Aspirant medical practitioners therefore 'train for uncertainty' (Fox 2000: 410), for example, through a process of intellectualization that entails the acquisition of greater knowledge and developing and applying methods for assessing probabilities to problems for which uncertainty exists. The ability to manage uncertainty is important for, 'in many situations, expressions of uncertainty by medical professionals would violate norms and invite punitive sanctions' (Adamson 1997: 135). Post-training physicians seek to increase control over clinical uncertainties through the assertion of individualized judgements made on the basis of personal experience, and by adopting particular treatment paradigms (Light 1979). Epistemological uncertainty can lead clinicians to be ambivalent towards diagnostic criteria, and flexible in their implementation of treatment protocols when faced with patient/parent resistance. Heteronomous values may therefore predominate (Elias 1974) as clinicians' interpretations and applications become, 'a far cry from how texts provide the confines for a diagnosis' (Rafalovich 2005: 306). Yair (2007: 689) argues that 'under conditions of uncertainty, doctors chose to conform – namely, to chose what others have elected – so as to gain social validation'. Critiques of biomedicine's (in)efficacy may have restricted the social influence of the profession in general, but as the media discourse of sports-related concussion shows, the challenge posed is relatively limited.

Uncertainty is also central to the patient-experience and may be manifest in unusual corporeal sensations, the inability to resolve a physical problem, and awareness of medical staff's epistemological and clinical uncertainties (Conrad 1987). Most significantly though, patients experience *existential uncertainty* – 'the individual's awareness that his or her future is open and undetermined' (Adamson 1997: 134). Existential uncertainty can include trajectory uncertainty (where recovery is unpredictable) and symptomatic uncertainty (where different symptoms occur at different times and in response to different stimuli), but primarily uncertainty over how illness may effect one's life more broadly. Existential uncertainty is central to the precarious and insecure careers of professional athletes and their typical coping mechanisms – (a) seeking second opinions; (b) negotiating the timing of surgery or other remedial action; (c) constructing 'treatment timetables' (Roderick 2006: 66) – give the athlete the feeling of progress and control over their recovery. Existential uncertainty has notable parallels with ideas about biographical disruption (Bury 1982, see Chapter 5) which in turn closely relate to illness narratives (Frank 1995, see Chapter 6). Existential uncertainty illustrates Elias's contention that in social contexts where events are unpredictable and high levels of insecurity are experienced, egocentric forms of knowledge increase in social valence (Elias 1987).

These concepts help to explain the experiences of concussion management described in interviews with healthcare professionals working in rugby union (2000–2001) and professional football (2014) (see Appendix). Despite the time lag between the studies, there is a high correlation between the two sets of findings. This can in part be explained by the fact that rugby union was at the forefront of concussion regulation, pioneering the precautionary policies now more widely adopted in sport. But additionally, and as much as the biomedical knowledge of concussion has developed, epistemological uncertainty over concussion remains rife and thus the contexts in which sports medicine clinicians attempt to manage head injuries have not fundamentally changed. Indeed, even the most recent consensus statement argues that 'the science of concussion is evolving' (McCrory *et al.* 2013: 250), and is punctuated by provisos and reservations, such as:

> 'conventional structural neuroimaging is typically normal in concussive injury'
> 'Brain CT (or MR Brain Scan) contributes little to concussion evaluation'
> 'alternative imaging technologies … are still at early stages of development'
> 'the significance of … genetic markers in the management of sports concussion risk or injury is unclear'
> how genetic and cytokine factors 'are affected in sporting concussion is not known'

'different electrophysiological recording techniques sometimes fail to differentiate between concussed athletes and controls'

Furthermore, it is noted that currently there is insufficient/limited evidence:

'to justify the routine use of (certain) biomarkers clinically'
'to recommend the widespread routine use of baseline neuropsychological testing'
'evaluating the effect of rest following sports-related concussion'
'that currently available protective equipment will prevent concussion'

This epistemological uncertainty feeds into clinical uncertainty and 'clinical and existential reactions to uncertainty play to and play off each other in all sorts of ways' (Adamson 1997: 154). In their everyday work settings (Freidson 1970) medical actors minimize conflict with their athlete-patients and adapt their medical knowledge and practice in order to enable relationships with coaches and players to remain functional. The constraint to make such 'compromises' constitutes the primary limitation to the medicalization of sport-related concussion.

Clinicians' experiences of managing concussion

The clinical uncertainty over concussion described in various media accounts was frequently and openly volunteered by the clinicians tasked with implementing concussion regulations. Clinicians typically described the condition as a 'huge grey area' (rugby doctor) or 'the difficult one' (football doctor). Interviewees sometimes rationalized their own uncertainty by preferring to use the less specific 'head injury' or responding to questions about concussion with questions of their own. A Premier League football physiotherapist, for instance, argued, 'If you're heading the ball is there a slight trauma to the brain? Then therefore is that concussion?... Is that a definition of it, or this, that and the other?' Clinicians also sought to legitimize their uncertainty by referring to the conditions under which they were required to practice, including assessing dehydrated players, the inability to clearly see what was happening on the pitch and, somewhat paradoxically, both the speed with which players can recover (mainly in football) and the pressures to quickly diagnose (mainly in rugby). Club doctors typically attempted to overcome clinical uncertainty through a process of investigation and intellectualization, exploring medical literature, talking to medical officers employed by the national governing body, or sending players to EM clinics. But attempts to alleviate clinical uncertainty are undermined by the epistemological uncertainty evident in the broader sports medicine community. For instance, a football doctor questioned the evidence for both the graduated RTP and the existence of second concussion syndrome, prophetically concluding 'so lots of uncertainty'.

Epistemological and clinical uncertainty intertwined with the injured athlete's existential uncertainty. Concussion injuries are unique not, as is often claimed, due to their invisibility but because the physical symptoms do not always (or even frequently) impair sporting performance on the pitch. For example, typically it was stated that 'you don't feel as though there is anything wrong with you' (rugby player). Concussed athletes therefore experience uncertainty because their bodies become dys-eased (Leder 1990), but they seldom experience problems that they themselves could not resolve and rarely, or only briefly, experienced uncertainty over their ability to function as normal. Thus, a football physiotherapist described the difficulties of conducting a graduated RTP: 'I've been challenged on that ... it's well "you know if he feels fine why can't he just train tomorrow"'. Such challenges ultimately shape their practice.

More particularly, a concussed player's existential uncertainty is unlikely to be relieved through consultation with a clinician because proscribed treatment simply entails physical and cognitive rest. Indeed, a concussed player's existential uncertainty is likely to *increase* as a consequence of a medical consultation because clinicians are required to impose periods of abstention from the game. This *will* produce uncertainties over team selection and, ultimately, questions about what the injury 'means' for a player's career. CISG make players' usual coping mechanisms redundant and so players are frequently reluctant to seek medical advice. For instance, a retired rugby player argued that, 'there have been times where both players and management have said, "avoid the possibility of seeing a doctor and being diagnosed". It's just a matter of keeping away'. Similarly, while a football physiotherapist argued, 'I'm sure they've [players] hidden symptoms in the past and again that's the complexity of concussion'. Thus, players' existential uncertainty arising from concussion symptoms leads them to be *less* rather than more dependent on clinicians, and heightens conflicts between clinicians and players and coaches (Malcolm 2009).

The convergence of these aspects of uncertainty serves to limit clinical management and thus the medicalization of sport-related concussions. Ultimately, clinicians de-professionalize their practice when they implement diagnostic and treatment guidelines in ways that serve to counteract, or minimize, patient non-compliance. A manifestation of this is the tendency to centre the definition of concussion upon LOC. Asked what symptoms were decisive, a football physiotherapist argued that 'I think LOC is. I think that would possibly dictate how much the severity of the initial trauma was'. Similarly, a rugby doctor noted, 'if someone is knocked out and there were signs of neurological disturbance, then I would *probably seriously think about* diagnosing concussion' (emphasis added). LOC had the advantage of not only being the most visible symptom, but also the most severe and the most widely accepted within the lay knowledge of the sports subculture. Clinicians ultimately adopt LOC as the basis for diagnosis because they prefer 'to be existentially secure in a supporting social group rather than being empirically correct in isolation' (Yair 2007: 687); they prioritize knowledge that 'works' in their everyday experience (Elias 1987).

Because this concession of definitive, expert knowledge ultimately threatens to undermine clinicians' authoritative status, they tend to invoke strategies that obscure their clinical uncertainty, re-assert their expertise and thus ensure their clients' continued reliance upon them. First, clinicians seek to avoid a specific diagnosis. In addition to using the most stringent and unequivocal criteria (LOC), clinicians referred to 'public concussions and keep-quiet concussions' (rugby doctor) and a reluctance to 'use the c-word' (rugby physiotherapist). A football physiotherapist described their stock response to a player complaining of concussion symptoms: 'I'm always like, "Do you want to have this conversation? As soon as you tell me you're dizzy…"'. Second, clinicians rationalized the use of their own experience to enable personal 'guidelines' to supersede standardized diagnostic protocols. Experiential knowledge included understanding how a player usually performed and considering whether a player could continue to withstand the impacts that playing would entail. As one rugby doctor argued, 'It's best not to diagnose it. It's best to have an opinion as to whether the player should be playing or not'. Finally, clinicians sought to individualize concussions and so remove diagnosis away from the necessarily generalized regulations. Clinicians therefore suggested that consideration of a player's recent injury history and/or knowledge of previous reactions to head injuries should inform an individual case management approach: 'you do notice a difference to somebody who is not right because if you're watching them, sometimes the loud ones are very quiet, sometimes they're just, I know it's not very scientific but, you know, they're not themselves' (football physiotherapist).

In contrast therefore to the medicalization of concussion evident at the conceptual and institutional levels, clinical actors and their identities are fundamentally problematized as they attempt to manage concussions in their everyday work settings. Bereft of institutional support in the form of epistemological certainty, questions about the appropriateness of their clinical practice lead to a variety of compromises including the rejection of medical understandings of concussion in favour of the adoption of lay knowledge which, ultimately, 'works' on a social and emotional level. The medicalization of concussion is therefore restricted due to an inability to deliver the social value promised by medicine, and the identities of clinical actors become less medically-rooted, and increasingly determined by lay influences.

Conclusion

This analysis of concussion in sport provides a salient reminder that medicine is not monolithic, but constructed of separate spheres which sometimes work at different levels and in contradictory ways. These differences only rarely surface but when they do they demonstrate the ease with which we can exaggerate medicine's social power. For instance, the critiques of existing concussion regulations revealed in interviews with clinicians were made rather more publicly by a senior Australian sports medicine doctor, John Orchard. Orchard suggested that potential responses to the application of new CISGs might be 'to rename [an injury], turn a blind eye, or pull players off who I would previously have been OK with playing and hurt the team's chances'. He thus argued that these policy developments would be seen by club doctors, 'as an unwelcome intrusion into their practice and a lack of confidence in their ability to properly manage players' (cited in Partridge 2014: 70). Similarly, despite overtly premised to the contrary, disputes have arisen in relation to the content and construction of so-called 'consensus' statements. Craton and Leslie (2014: 93) for instance, point to a 'lack of diagnostic specificity, management strategies that are not evidence based, and rehabilitation goals that are not attainable'. Specifically, they note that: the inclusion criteria for diagnosis are too broad and therefore could capture multiple other conditions; there is no supportive evidence for prescribing physical and cognitive rest (the latter being a highly problematic concept anyway); and relying on the notion of 'asymptomatic' to guide graduated RTP is not operational, as most people are never fully asymptomatic of the inclusion criteria.

These epistemological debates fuel a growing chorus of criticism at what are perceived to be inherent conflicts of interest (Craton and Leslie 2014). For instance, a comparison of contributors to the various concussion statements shows the emergence of a 'closed shop', dominated by employees of sports federations, player associations and companies that sell diagnostic and evaluative equipment. It has been argued that there is insufficient transparency in: (a) the burden of proof and the level of agreement required for 'consensus' to be achieved; (b) the conduct of proceedings; and (c) the selection of panel members, and thus one 'may reasonably ask whether the consensus is the outcome of predetermined selection rather than the conformity of scientific opinion' (McNamee et al. 2015: 198). Moreover, the sponsorship of this process by sports governing bodies 'could be seen as an attempt to steer the concussion agenda' and may ultimately result in the production of guidelines 'simply used to justify their own policies and practices' (McNamee et al. 2015: 194). As Bercovitz (2000: 25) argues, consensus statements 'may be regarded as more a reflection of the desire of selected "experts" and scientists to impose their worldview on research and practice'. As we have seen, the views and interests of this faction within sport medicine do not necessarily accord with those of the clinicians tasked with the day-to-day management of concussion in sport, but their prominence is such that they have largely persuaded the (sports) media of the value, if not *necessity*, of increasing medical regulation of this sporting/social issue.

Despite internal divisions within (sports) medicine, it is notable that a manifest outcome of changing concussion policy has been to consolidate medical control over this social issue. For instance, the most recent concussion assessment tool, SCAT 3, identifies physicians as the appropriate professionals to take responsibility for concussion management and thus disregards the probable greater experience of physiotherapists in dealing with head injuries. A series of changes to the CISG have reinforced this, as the initial recommendation for the medical management of players exhibiting *any* symptoms has been superseded by the less conservative emphasis on medical intervention when cases of concussion have explicitly been *diagnosed*. Importantly, the former was essentially amenable to lay assessment while the later places concussion within a domain that has traditionally been the basis of medicine's authoritative status (Jutel 2009). The implementation of such guidelines further shifts the balance of jurisdictional duties between first aiders/sports trainers and physicians. Partridge (2014) notes that AFL and NRL regulations require players suspected of sustaining a concussion to be assessed by a first aider yet also that players 'need an urgent medical assessment by a medical practitioner' because 'the management of head injury is difficult for non-medical personnel' (Partridge 2014: 67, 68). Most fundamentally, however, the primacy of medicine is established by the continued provision in the CISG of all RTP decisions remaining 'largely in the realm of clinical judgment on an individual basis' (cited in McNamee *et al.* 2015: 192). Sports administrators may demonstrate a degree of reluctance to alter the structure and form of the pastime and product they see it as their duty to protect, and indeed sports medicine is notably deferential in this respect, but the medicalization of concussion (conceptually) is fuelled by support from the media and (in the US) legal institutions. Remarkably this jurisdictional expansion has occurred in relation to a condition that does not require esoteric skills or particularly specialist knowledge. The symptoms of concussion – memory loss, dizziness, loss of consciousness – are not hard to detect, although ironically the condition is now claimed to be, 'considered among the most complex injuries in sports medicine to diagnose, assess and manage' (McCrory *et al.* 2013: 7). Concussion, if it is difficult to diagnose, is so as a result of the medicalization of the condition.

In concluding this chapter, we should focus on the self-perpetuating nature of medicalization. When concerns about head injuries led to greater epidemiological exploration, biomedical research served to reinforce perceptions that concussion was both a serious social concern, and that it probably occurred more frequently than previously thought. This in turn generated the desire and provided the empirical support for increased regulation, which logically led to increased incidence, greater media exposure, heightened public concern and calls for further regulation. While the 2000–2001 research with elite rugby players revealed that just 25% had ever been formally diagnosed with concussion (Malcolm 2009), more recent research estimates that 50% of players are concussed *every* season (Fraas *et al.* 2013). While five years ago a professional footballer in England could RTP a few minutes after losing consciousness, now a player should be removed from play if there is 'any suspicion' (FA 2015: 542). While it would be irresponsible to suggest that concussion in sport is not worthy of further investigation it is difficult to see this 'concussion industry' (McNamee and Partridge 2013: 17) reversing and concussion becoming de-medicalized. Further biomedical research will almost inevitably uncover greater cause for concern in the future.

Such jurisdictional expansion invokes fundamental ethical questions about the autonomy of the individual athlete-patient. While cognizant of debates about how 'freely' such choices can be made within the sports subculture, athletes consistently and effectively resist regulation. A major impetus for these developments appears to a desire to uphold the (fundamentally flawed) sport–health ideology. We expand on these ideas in Chapter 10 where we explore the implementation of cardiac screening in sport.

Note

1 A further and fundamental problem with these regulations is their inherently contradictory advice. In addition to the provision of a head injury bin, the regulations state that players 'MUST NOT resume play once removed from the field for *suspected* concussion' (italics added). It is difficult to see how a player could undergo a head injury assessment if concussion was not suspected, thereby making the option to re-enter the field redundant.

Chapter 10

Medicalization and cardiac screening

As noted in Chapter 1, the screening of participants is another prominent manifestation of the medicalization of sport and consequently the focus of this book's penultimate chapter. Broadly speaking, medicine has been called upon to test participants' gender, use of performance-enhancing drugs or techniques and, in the case of Paralympic athletes, physical ability. The rationale for each of these programmes is essentially to safeguard equality for participants. In this respect the programmes differ from the way screening is more commonly understood in the sociology of medicine; namely, 'the purposeful application of tests to an asymptomatic population in order to classify people into those who are *unlikely* to have or develop a disease and those who are *likely* to have or develop a disease' (Armstrong and Eborall 2012: 162, emphasis in the original). However, all forms of screening are similarly influenced by social and political factors, and have ethical implications related to individual autonomy. Before considering the expansion of medical surveillance in sport through cardiac screening programmes, we briefly consider the multiple forms of medical screening to which sports participants are subject.

The first medical involvement in the sex segregation of sport was a test (of unspecified form) that took place at the 1936 Berlin Olympics after (false) accusations that the American sprinter Helen Stephens was a man. From 1948 the IOC required medical certification of 'female' participants' sex, while 'systematic, at-event, standardized, scientific sex tests' (Heggie 2010b: 159) were introduced at the Commonwealth Games and European Athletics Championship of 1966 and 'managed to keep out six who were hermaphrodites' and 'frighten the doubtful ones away' from the latter (IAAF President David [Lord Exeter] Burghley, cited in Wrynn 2004: 221). Fuelled by Western concerns about deviant Eastern European practices, in 1967 the IOC replaced these visual-cum-physical examinations with the Barr Body chromosome test. However, problems with the accuracy of this buccal smear test (chromosomal sex is not necessarily compatible with physiological or phenotypic sex) and in particular the successful appeal against a positive test by Maria Martinez-Patino, led to the adoption in

1992 of a test for a single gene found in the Y chromosome. Again this proved unreliable; for example eight people who 'failed' this test were allowed to compete in women's events at the 1996 Atlanta Olympics (Heggie 2010b). Most recently the IOC's (2003) Stockholm Consensus, which outlines the conditions for the participation of transsexuals, has been subject to criticism (Cavanaugh and Sykes 2006) and the IAAF and IOC's hyperandrogenism regulations, which require female athletes with certain hormonal profiles to undergo medical interventions, have been legally challenged on the ground of discrimination (BBC 2015c).

Screening for drug use was also introduced in the mid-1960s at the height of the Cold War. From the late 1980s, in-competition urine tests were gradually supplemented with out-of-competition-testing and from 2004 a 'whereabouts' system was introduced under which athletes must provide notification of their movements so that they can be tested at any time and at minimal notice. There have been trails of blood testing and 'biological passports' (where an athlete's data are compared over time to detect physiological changes) but this form of screening has been dogged by: (a) questions of fairness, including claims that it only identifies a tiny minority of illegal substance abuse (Waddington and Smith 2009); (b) concerns that testing benefits those with access to the most sophisticated and thus least detectable drugs; and (c) the suspicion (raised recently against Jamaica and Kenya, and verified in the case of Russia) that some athletes receive state support to evade detection. It is also questionable whether the exacting demands infringe athletes' liberties, with the system compared to the self-disciplinary mechanisms of the Foucauldian panopticon (Park 2005) and a Deleuzian surveillance system of technological and informational networks (Sluggett 2011). While both seem to exaggerate the degree of athlete compliance (most analysts believe drug use is endemic in elite sport), the subjects of these testing regimes have little trust in the reliability of testing, find the whereabouts system punitive (Overbye and Wagner 2013), and report psychological responses that include fear, stress and perceived violations of privacy and personal integrity (Elbe and Overbye 2013).

The organization of sport for athletes with disabilities is similarly predicated on the medical classification of participants. Events have traditionally been based on a disability-specific classification which, a priori, is initiated by medical diagnosis but, in an attempt to create conditions of fairness, athletes are further categorized into groups which reflect *the degree* of impairment. Pressure to make the Paralympics both more organizationally manageable and commercially marketable have led to a contraction in the number of athlete categories, with the introduction of an 'integrated functional classification system' (which eschews disability grouping and focuses on an individuals' range of motion, muscular strength and limb coordination) or a system in which athletes with various disabilities compete together, but are assigned a kind of multiplier which converts the individuals' performances into a points value by which participants are ranked (Howe and Jones 2006). Changes to the classificatory system have impacted greatest on the most severely disabled and thus this has disempowered the Paralympic practice community.

However, in many ways the testing programme most central to the medicalization of sport has been cardiac screening. For example, it was cardiac research, in response to parents' anxieties about the effects of vigorous exercise on children, which led to the formation of the ACSM (see Chapter 3). Indeed the identity of sports medicine as a medical specialism has been fundamentally linked to changing perceptions of the relationship between exercise and the pathology/physiology of the heart. What Heggie (2009) calls 'a century of cardiomythology' resulted in the identification of 'athlete's heart' (enlarged and slow beating) as a normal consequence of extreme levels of physical activity. Data from electrocardiogram (ECG) testing at the 1958 Commonwealth Games showed that 'the normal body, and normal readings from medical technology, were no longer appropriate measures for the athletic body' (Heggie 2009: 289), and so fuelled the emergence of a *sports* medicine specialism to treat this physiologically distinct demographic group/clinical object. Paradoxically and problematically, in light of the sport–health ideology, exercise alters the heart in ways that 'overlap with disease phenotypes' (Chandra *et al.* 2012: 1).

However, while publicity over the aforementioned forms of screening largely revolves around notions of cheating, the increasing public profile of cardiac screening in sport speaks directly to the sport–health ideology. Widely publicized incidents in recent years include the sudden cardiac death (SCD) of footballer Marc Vivien Defoe during the 2003 Confederations Cup, two Belgian footballers within a fortnight of each other in the spring of 2015 (BBC 2015d), and Patrick Ekeng while playing for Dinamo Bucharest in 2016 (BBC 2016). Non-elite athletes have similarly been affected, such as Kris Cook and David Seath, participants in the 2014 RideLondon public cycling event and 2016 London Marathon respectively (BBC 2014; Gani 2016). SCD represents an acute social issue and thus an ideal opportunity for medicine to expand its domain of influence in sport.

This chapter explores the policy responses of sports governing bodies and the subjective experiences of athletes who have taken part in screening programmes. It examines the principles of a sociological analysis of screening followed by the rationale for the implementation of screening in sport. Following a discussion of footballers' experiences of the process, it explicates the social construction of the medical knowledge underpinning such screening programmes. It concludes that the existence and persistence of this form of medicalization – that is to say, the medical surveillance (Armstrong 1995) of the athlete population – ultimately depends upon the significance of the sport–health ideology.

The rationale for cardiac screening in sport

Medical screening for early disease detection normally consists of four stages. Initially, a population is identified as sufficiently at risk to merit preventative attention. Candidates are then invited to undergo biomedical or other tests which are used to (re-)calculate an individual's risk, before more detailed tests are offered to a sub-section of those initially screened. Ultimately, the purpose is to offer medical interventions (Heyman 2010). Because implementation is often contentious – as the examples in the introductory section suggest – a 1960s WHO-commissioned report sought to establish criteria that have since become a 'public health classic' (Andermann *et al*. 2008: 317) and 'the gold standard for initiating a population-screening programme' (Timmermans and Buchbinder 2012: 208). But while Wilson and Jungner's (1968) *Principles and Practice of Screening for Disease* are widely cited by medical researchers, sociologists and, now, sports organizations, 'there seems no generally accepted way of using these principles, or derived criteria, as objective decision tools' (Pollit 2006, cited in Andermann *et al*. 2008: 318). Debates in sport replicate these disagreements for, while Papadakis *et al*. (2008: 810) argue that cardiac screening 'does not fulfil most of the WHO criteria', Corrado *et al*. (2011: 943) state that it meets 'the most important' ones. The aim of this section is to review the literature on cardiac screening in sport in light of Wilson and Jungner's principles of screening (see Box 10.1) in order to evaluate the rationale for implementation.

First, while researchers generally identify SCD in young athletes as an important health problem, there is considerable disagreement over how important an issue it is. This issue returns us to the concepts of

---

Box 10.1 The principles of screening

The condition sought should be an important health problem
There should be an accepted treatment for patients
Facilities for diagnosis and treatment should be available
There should be a recognizable latent or early symptomatic stage
There should be a suitable test or examination
The test should be acceptable to the population
The natural history of the condition should be adequately understood
There should be an agreed policy on whom to treat as patients
The cost of case finding should be economically balanced in relation to other medical care demands
Case finding should be a continuing process and not a 'once and for all' project

Source: Wilson and Jungner (1968).

epistemological and clinical uncertainty discussed in Chapter 9. For instance, the UK charity Cardiac Risk in the Young (CRY), estimates that the risk of SCD in athletes is around 1:50,000, the British Heart Foundation (BHF 2013) estimates the figure to lie between this and 1:100,000, and Papadakis *et al.* (2008) report an incidence as low as 0.5 per 100,000 in one study. Uncertainty over the frequency and thus social significance of sport-related SCD is compounded by the variance of demographic groups employed in research samples. Older and disproportionately male cohorts produce higher rates (Corrado *et al.* 2011). Moreover although being an athlete is said to increase one's risk of SCD by a factor of 2.8 (Ljungqvist *et al.* 2009: 6), there is no consensus over what level of sporting activity increases risk (and by how much). There have been no randomized control trials of screening because these are 'ethically and technically challenging' (Elston and Stein 2011: 576), 'difficult or impossible to deliver' (Heyman 2010: 4). Indicative of the confusion, Whyte and Wilson have called for 'an international embargo on guessing the incidence of sudden death' (Hamilton *et al.* 2012: i10–11).

Epistemological and clinical uncertainty is common in screening for heart conditions. For instance, Daly (1989) found that, because clinicians frequently used other criteria to interpret technological evaluations, 'the choice of cardiologist may be a more certain determinant of the diagnosis than the patient's anatomy' (Daly 1989: 109). Lutfey and McKinlay (2009) concur. Because the diagnosis of Chronic Heart Disease (CHD) is relatively uncertain, doctors frequently have to consider alternatives (such as gastro-intestinal or mental health issues), and in so doing invariably pick up on other cues, which may be physiological (the patient 'looks' ill) or social (how families might positively or negatively influence patient perception). However, these problems are compounded in sport-related screening, which is 'an attempt to detect a cluster of conditions with a common potential outcome, rather than one single condition' (Anderson *et al.* 2012: 331). Consequently there are disagreements over what constitutes a suitable test and who should be treated as a patient. Basic screening programmes entail the self-reporting of symptoms and family history (often via a questionnaire), and a physical examination. Alternative programmes supplement these with a 12 lead ECG, echocardiogram (ECHO), stress tests, Holter monitoring and/or imaging methods such as a cardiac MRI or CT angiography (Borjesson and Crezner 2012).

Deployment of these tests varies across nation-states as well as between and within sports. For instance, the AHA and ACC recommend self-reporting and physical examination but not the routine use of ECGs for athletes at any level. Conversely, the Consensus Statement of the European Society of Cardiology (ESC) calls for the mandatory ECG screening of athlete populations (Corrado *et al.* 2005). Correlatively, no mass ECG screening programme has (yet) been instituted in the US, while ECGs are the norm throughout Europe. Frequently cited as an exemplar, Italy's mandatory annual screening (consisting of a self-report questionnaire, physical examination, ECG and exercise stress test) incorporates minor level athletes and secondary school pupils (Hillis *et al.* 2011). Luxembourg, Poland and Greece screen all 'competitive' athletes' while in France, Germany, Sweden and the Netherlands compulsory screening is confined to those defined as high performance athletes (Corrado *et al.* 2011). However, in Britain there is no state supported screening programme and the BHF (2013) explicitly rejects publicly-funded screening of professional athletes and only supports targeted testing where family history suggests a high risk of inherited cardiac disease. Consequently the implementation of cardiac screening is a culturally specific process.

The IOC position is outlined in the Lausanne Recommendations (Bille 2006). This *recommends* cardiac screening (history, physical exam and ECG) of all participants up to 35 years old, but defers to international sports federations regarding the specifics of implementation. Consequently, considerable variation exists between sports. For example, the IAAF (2012) *recommend* that athletes are physically examined prior to participation in major international competitions, while FIFA *recommend* that footballers have a physical examination and ECG test every two years. Further differences exist within sports. For instance, UEFA operates *mandatory* screening for participants in each of its national and club competitions. Similarly, the IRB (n.d.) state that geographic, economic, social and medical differences between members and across different levels of the game necessitate tiered implementation. Consequently for recreational players the IRB recommends (as a minimum) the biennial use of a screening questionnaire for players up to 20 years old, that professional clubs and all national/multi-national tournaments should supplement this with an ECG 'if logistically possible', and that a questionnaire and physical examination '*must* be completed on all players prior to participation' in IRB-managed competitions (emphasis added). Preferably, but not necessarily, this should be supplemented by an ECG, 'interpreted by a medical practitioner experienced in reading sports ECG'. As Müller (2012: 286, emphasis in the original) concludes, 'the current PPS [pre-participation screening] *standard* is that there is no *standard*'.

Finally, it can be seen that the penultimate principle of Wilson and Jungner's (1968) criteria – the cost of case finding relative to other potential health interventions – is also contentious. Debates over the economic justification for cardiac screening in sport are influenced by questions about the type of screening and the subject population. Borjesson and Crezner (2012: i5) surmise that screening based on history and physical examination 'requires significant cost … but with a low yield of disease detection', that ECG-screening has economic benefits equivalent to many other accepted forms of screening, and that the use of ECHO comes at a very high cost for a small increase in sensitivity. Moreover, the estimated costs of ECG screening vary widely – from €36 per athlete in Italy, to $374 in the USA – presumably due to the economies of scale in Italy where screening is extensively implemented. While at the elite level it is clearly feasible for professional teams to periodically screen all players using an ECG (and indeed ECHO), many advocates of cardiac screening for competitive athletes recognize that, 'a national screening programme to detect silent cardiac diseases in athletes cannot be regarded as cost effective' (Papadakis *et al.* 2008: 810).

Ultimately, assessment of whether 'the overall benefits of the programme … outweigh the harm' (Andermann *et al.* 2008: 318), depends on estimates of the balance between accurate detection and the iatrogenic costs of false negative and false positive results. The IRB state that between 15 and 30% of athletes suffering SCD 'will not be identified even with intensive cardiac screening' (IRB n.d.), and Sanjay Sharma, a leading cardiologist and founder of CRY, states that 'an ECG picks up around 60 to 70 per cent of cases' (quoted in Coghlan 2012). Papadakis *et al.* (2008) illustrate a further complication in estimating iatrogenic costs by noting different rates of detection for different conditions. They estimate that ECG abnormalities are 'exhibited by 95% of people with hypertrophic cardiomyopathy (HCM) and 80% of those with arrhythmogenic right ventricular cardiomyopathy', resulting in a false-negative rate of 5% and 20% respectively. Corrado *et al.* (2011) estimate that ECG testing is 87% accurate and thus compares favourably with personal history and physical examination (less than 10% accurate) but unfavourably with an ECHO (claimed to be 100% accurate).

While ECG-based screening is thought to lead to relatively few false-negatives, it produces a significant number of false-positives. For example, 9% of a 42,000 Italian population screening programme had positive ECG findings and further examination led 2% of the population to be diagnosed with cardiovascular disorders and 0.2% to be disqualified from sport (Corrado *et al.* 2011). This equates to 2940 and 3706 false-positives respectively. In a study of nearly 2000 NFL athletes, the entire 25% found to have ECG abnormalities were false-positives (Magalski *et al.* 2008). Elston and Stein (2011) estimate that a UK-wide ECG-based screening programme of 1.5 million young athletes would produce 140,000 referrals, 31,522 disqualifications from sport, and prevent just 40 SCDs per year.

While 'there appears to be a general truth that predictive accuracy has to be traded against economic and iatrogenic costs' (Heyman 2010: 3) the 'cost' of a false-positive from cardiac screening in sport has distinct elements. Prohibition from sport might have negative psychological and physiological consequences (Menafoglio *et al.* 2013) but could also terminate a highly lucrative career. This was highlighted in the case of the Italian swimmer and Olympic gold medallist, Domenico Fioravanti, who contested the decision to ban him from the sport after a diagnosis of HCM (Müller 2012). In sympathy with such cases, opponents of more comprehensive and particularly mandatory screening regimes base their opposition on the medical ethical principle, 'first do no harm' (Hamilton *et al.* 2012: i11).

In conclusion, it has long been accepted that while 'the central idea of early disease detection and treatment is essentially simple … the path to its successful achievement [is difficult]' (Wilson and Jungner 1968, cited in Andermann *et al.* 2008). However, the rationale for cardiac screening in sport at either elite or population levels, whether voluntary or mandatory, appears far from compelling. In the next section, we explore Wilson and Jungner's sixth principle – that a test should be acceptable to the population – as part of a discussion of the procedures used and the experiences of those in professional football who have either been subjected to, or charged with the implementation of, cardiac screening (see Appendix for a discussion of the research projects in which this data was generated).

Who wants screening? The experiences of footballers and clinicians

The Muamba incident led the FA's Chief Medical Officer to clarify existing policy through various media. This revealed that ECG-based cardiac screening, funded by the Professional Footballers Association (PFA), was 'offered' to approximately 800 young (16–18) footballers per year as they enter the academies of professional clubs, and that subsequently 'one or two [per year] are advised to give up football' (BBC 2012). Additionally, cardiac screening is mandatory for players selected to train or play for all English representative sides, and the FA recommends that players are screened every two years in accordance with FIFA recommendations (Scott, Andy 2012). However, as we have seen in relation to clinical appointments and the management of head injuries, implementation of FA medical regulations is somewhat sporadic. Most clinicians from the lower divisions said that the PFA-funded programme was effectively the only screening that occurred. As one physiotherapist said, 'unfortunately we get into the sort of mind that if it's not compulsory then why do we need to do it?' There was a perception that clubs in the higher divisions screened more frequently, but interviewees who were clinicians at bigger clubs indicated that the greater frequency was largely a consequence of their players' being screened in relation to UEFA and FIFA competitions. The fact that, in practice, clubs screen players as *in*frequently as possible, aligns with what we have seen in terms of the culture of sport being relatively resistant to medical input and thus acting as a barrier to medicalization.

The expansion of medical jurisdictional boundaries and the impact of screening on recipient populations are central to medical sociological analyses of the practice. Key issues identified include: (i) considerations of informed consent and the (sometimes) high rates of non-compliance to screening initiatives; (ii) the psychological impact of screening including the anxiety experienced from being invited to have (and/or subsequently undergoing) a test, the impact of diagnosis, the uncertainty associated with a false-positive result; (iii) the potential for coercion through such population surveillance; and (iv) the consequences of blurring the health/illness dichotomy through the creation of an 'at risk' population (Armstrong and Eborall 2012). Studies have further illustrated how lay perspectives influence subjects' responses to the screening process. Subjects may not understand the nature of the test or the choices available, and so cannot give informed consent to the procedure (Pilnick 2008). Where they do, a variety of non-medical factors (such as personal cost, modesty, resistance to authority) and notions of candidacy (an individual's assessments of their own risk) may mediate responses to being identified as an at risk population (Pfeffer 2004). This can lead to lay contestation of medical expert knowledge (Armstrong 2005). Daly's (1989) fourfold typology of patients who undergo cardiac screening (*worried*; *distracted*; *athletic* and *other*) is particularly pertinent here, as the *athletic* were identified as the group most likely to resist the 'illness' label, be sceptical of medical advice and deny or challenge the diagnosis. Such challenges to medicalization stem from the disjuncture between medical evaluation and patients' embodied experiences. How then is cardiac screening experienced in English professional football?

Given the variable implementation, it was perhaps predictable that interviews would reveal a widespread misunderstanding of FA regulations. For example, all clinicians suggested that testing was mandatory for (as opposed to offered to) apprentices. Players' comments also revealed their lack of understanding of the process to which they were subject. Rarely did interviewees describe being given information to read prior to the test and some accounts revealed confusion over the purpose of such tests (cf. Pilnick 2008). Often (though not always) interviewees were aware that their parents/guardians had signed to give consent, but this did not translate to their own understanding: 'my mum was with me at the time ... I didn't have clue' (academy footballer).

While, according to FA regulations, screening should not have appeared mandatory (the exception seems to be in relation to selection a national team), most footballers were either simply summonsed or made an offer that effectively coerces the individual to undergo cardiac screening (Anderson *et al.* 2012). Recalling being tested in the aftermath of the Muamba incident, one player stated:

> they told us we had to get it done because it was after the Muamba thing. So it was, kind of, compulsory that we had to get it done ... everybody else was going to do it and I'd be the only one not doing it

... every day they brought that [Muamba] up.... So you can't really say, 'no I'm not doing it'.

Most players, like the subjects of other screening programmes (e.g. Daly 1989), were compliant – 'happy for the club to do that' (academy footballer) – and didn't feel the need to ask questions about the purpose or process. Interviewees trusted their employer's medical provision simply because they were a professional football club and thus assumed to have the best available equipment. Although they reported experiencing anxiety – 'it could be the end of your career, so I was kind of scared ... I was kind of nervous' – there was a sense, *pace* Howson (1999), that participation in screening was the morally responsible thing to do. As one apprentice footballer argued, 'I had no choice actually. I had to do it because it's important to you because you never know'.

But in considering their likely responses to a positive result, apprentices shed a different light on the acceptability of the screening process to them for, perhaps not surprisingly, they exhibited similar resistance and noncompliance to 'positive' screening outcomes as the 'athletic' group of cardiac patients identified by Daly (1989). A player whose first test was inconclusive continued to train as normal despite being told 'there might be something wrong'. When others considered how they might react to the discovery of an underlying cardiac problem, they envisaged being 'heartbroken.... But I think I'd still carry on. I wouldn't give up what I do'. Another, when asked how he might respond to a positive test highlighted the problems of the disjuncture between technical readings and the embodied experience of feeling healthy and fit: 'like I love football, I can't stop football. Even if my heart has a problem but I'm feeling good I don't think I would stop football'.

Clinicians' experiences of dealing with abnormal findings confirmed what the players suggested about the acceptability of such tests. Where screening results posed existential uncertainties for players – in particular where screening results threatened a player with retirement – invariably the response was to dispute or negotiate the precautionary medical advice. One physiotherapist described how an apprentice was allowed (albeit following discussions with a cardiac consultant) to postpone surgery 'just so he had enough time to take him all the way up to the end of the season to give him the best possible chance of getting a professional contract'. Another recalled an apprentice who appealed against a club's decision to release him claiming that he could not be insured. The FA medical committee, following two further cardiac assessments, upheld the club's position. The player was 'absolutely, yes, devastated ... [it] absolutely dumbfounded him' (physiotherapist). At other times the players were successful in getting their wish to carry on. A third physiotherapist described the situation in which a player with a longstanding cardiac issue 'used to have to sign a waiver every season to say "I understand the risks" '. A club doctor recalled that, in his 20-year career, two players had been advised to cease playing, but that both had elected to carry on. Both had completed their careers without incident indicating ultimately false positive results.

Such experiences led one clinician to question the ethics of the screening programme:

> what's the morality of doing it? And you know, if you have to sit a player down and go 'you have got significant cardiac [conditions]' and you know the player is going to have to retire off it, and they may never have an issue. It's a strange one isn't it?

This physiotherapist went on to point to the uncertainty of the prognosis as problematic, 'what do you do?... [say] "you can go out and play with your mates, but you can't play in an academy game". It's a bit strange isn't it?... I mean how many people walking around have an issue?'

Behind this potential and actual non-compliance lay players' notions of candidacy (Pfeffer 2004). Perceptions of candidacy (or lay evaluations of risk) are both widespread amongst screened populations and exacerbated by the specific way in which risk is employed in relation to cardiac screening in football. Interviewees (both players and clinicians) revealed that the feedback from cardiac screening in football was confined to a 'yes–no' or 'normal–abnormal' reading. No interviewee had been given feedback in terms of a quantified risk assessment. One player who had been given more information on the test results noted, 'they said you have a genetic type of thing but it's not serious, everything's all right'. Another player recalled asking the physiotherapist for his test results, 'and he goes "yes, everything's spot on" '.

In the absence of a quantitative risk assessment and in the knowledge, post-Muamba, of the limitations of screening, players envisage their own candidacy of SCD as largely a matter of luck. One player, for instance, argued that, 'it could happen to anyone at any time', while another stated that 'It just happens, it's just life, isn't it?... Yeah it's just luck'. They therefore undertake a somewhat passive 'personalised and individual consideration of risk' (Armstrong 2005: 174). But, fundamentally, it is the test (i.e. the medicalization of sport) that *generates* risk for the subject (Saukko *et al.* 2012). Insurance companies do not require footballers to have cardiac screening prior to taking out a policy (James 2012); however, as the above example shows, such companies may refuse cover to those who present abnormal findings. Consequently, for most players the impact of screening is at best benign and at worst unwelcome. Consequently, like the forms of screening discussed in the introduction to this chapter, athletes can and do seek to 'conceal symptoms, or mitigate them' for fear of discovering diseases that will harm their sports careers (Menafoglio *et al.* 2013: 13).

In light of the ambiguity in the rationale for cardiac screening in sport, and data on the process and experiences of cardiac screening – which seem to indicate that such test are, in practice, not wholly acceptable to athlete recipients and in some respects their sports club employers – the existence of cardiac screening in sport must stem from the broader social and political dimensions of the process. In the final section we explore how medical discourse about cardiac screening in sport augments an essentially biological explanation of what is, a priori, a lifestyle-influenced condition. Moreover, in assessing the outcomes of the implementation of screening, we see the self-perpetuating character of screening programmes and thus the force of medicalization processes.

Cardiac screening, the social construction of medical knowledge and medicalization

Ironically, given that by definition the cardiac screening of athletes implies that lifestyle is a significant contributory factor, the consensus view amongst clinicians and sports administrators is that cardiac problems manifest in young athletes essentially stem from biological factors. Typically, exercise is described as merely 'the trigger' (Corrado *et al.* 2011: 936) which correlatively means that it can be argued that, 'sport is not per se the cause of the greater incidence of SCD' (Ljungqvist *et al.* 2009: 6). If this were true there could be no rationale for solely screening the elite and not all who take part in sport. The position is all the more problematic given that it is well established that exercise alters the appearance and structure of the heart and, as illustrated above, that there are so many uncertainties in relation to screening programmes designed to detect underlying cardiac problems in young athletes.

These caveats signal the relevance of the broader political and social aspects of cardiac screening in sport. The way certain debates are framed, especially those related to the screening of different demographic groups, lead the impact of lifestyle on SCD to be consistently underplayed or ignored. Moreover, as screening programmes necessarily produce knowledge which alters the understanding of the conditions for which they test, they tend to fuel the momentum of medicalization by pathologizing the athletic population and producing evidence that justifies the perpetuation of further screening. Thus, screening as a form of medicalization through surveillance is likely to become increasingly widespread (Timmermans and Buchbinder 2012).

As noted earlier it is doubtful that RCTs for screening (in sport) could ever be meaningfully conducted. Consequently, knowledge about cardiac health and the impact of screening is largely derived from screening programmes themselves. As Timmermans and Buchbinder (2012: 209) note 'any prior understanding of disease is inevitably found to be insufficient once population screening is instituted'. For example, Menafoglio *et al.* (2013) discuss changes in the ESC criteria for reading ECG results in athletes, with recommendations revised in 2010 to reduce the frequency of positive tests. These new criteria, however, resulted in highly varied results 'likely explained by a variable adherence to the ESC criteria on the basis of ... local experience' (Menafoglio *et al.* 2013: 16) and consequently the authors advocated adoption of new, more restrictive, criteria which provide 'the best balance between sensitivity and specificity' (Menafoglio *et al.* 2013: 18). It is, of course, the duty of researchers and clinicians to engage in a continual process of procedural refinement, but in the case of (cardiac) screening this fine-tuning fundamentally impacts on the rationale for existing programmes. Specifically, these changes, it is claimed, will limit 'costs, anxiety and inappropriate diagnoses' (Menafoglio *et al.* 2013: 18). However, regardless of how conservatively diagnostic criteria are applied, the generation of an 'at risk' and therefore pathologized population is an inherent feature of all screening programmes (Saukko *et al.* 2012). Hence 'the knowledge generated affects the rationale for population-based screening', and it is very rare for such new knowledge to 'turn back the screening momentum' (Timmermans and Buchbinder 2012: 210).

The 'bridging work' of clinicians who, through screening, encounter anomalies in understanding, also plays a key role in sustaining screening programmes. Clinicians undertake 'bridging work ... to reconcile the promise of technology with the realities of implementation' (Timmermans and Buchbinder 2012: 208). In so doing they reinforce paradigmatic assumptions (e.g. of physiological rather than social causation) and thus centre medicine in illness resolution. Mirroring the findings of previous studies (e.g. Daly 1989), clinician interviewees gave widely varying estimates of the frequency with which they encountered positive screening tests, thus indicating that relatively subjective individual judgements are fundamental to diagnosis. For example, two Premiership clubs clinicians, both of whom had been in post for over 10 years, described problematic outcomes as infrequent (encountered never and just once respectively), while physiotherapists in the lower divisions described the prevalence as '10–15%', '5–10%' and 'four in four years'. Another noted that while 'the majority come back with issues in terms of looking at ... it will just say "lightly athletic heart" with recommended repeat annual screening'; that is to say, continued medical surveillance. Underscoring the variability of the testing procedure, one physiotherapist noted that, 'when we had the screenings done last year the cardiologist pretty much sent everyone back for a cardiac MRI ... [It transpired that] the family histories hadn't been sent back so they all, they were all actually OK'.

Wider contextual factors also impact on diagnosis (Lutfey and McKinlay 2009). A doctor discussed how the pressures of transfer deadlines led clinicians to consider evidence (physiological but also historical/social) from beyond the data generated during pre-signing medicals:

> On transfer deadline day the player can be coming in two or three hours prior to the deadline and you have to do an ECG and make a decision. So it's a case of knowing. Of course on the face of it some of them look awful but in fact they're not.

Screening therefore is not solely about disease detection, but becomes a form of scientific data gathering through which diseases/conditions 'ontologically and epistemology [change] what we understand as a specific disease and how we know about a disease' (Timmermans and Buchbinder 2012: 210). Although interviewees did not reveal the same level or dynamics of uncertainty that they did in relation to concussion (see Chapter 9), it is reasonable to assume that their everyday work is contoured by similar concerns to protect their professional identities and remain socially useful.

Because screening programmes generate new and self-fulfilling information, and 'bridge work' shapes the anomalies that might detract from its 'usefulness', screening data occupy a privileged epistemological position. For example, one of the most frequently cited studies in this area analysed the annual incidence of SCD in the Veneto region of Italy from 1979 to 2004, and concluded that cases fell by 89% as a consequence of the introduction of population screening (Corrado et al. 2011: 937). These findings have recently been questioned by researchers exploring the impact of an Israeli mandatory ECG-based screening programme introduced in 1997. Steinvil et al. (2011) undertook a media content analysis over a 25-year period and identified a total of 24 cases of SCD, 11 before and 13 after the implementation of screening. When weighted to allow for changes in sports participation, this equates to an *increase* in incidence of SCD from 2.54 to 2.66 per 100,000 person-years. The authors conclude, therefore, that the policy 'had no apparent influence on the incidence of sudden death in athletes' in Israel (Steinvil et al. 2011: 1293). Moreover, the authors further claim that had they compared post-implementation rates with SCD rates in the two years prior to implementation (as the Veneto study did), they would have shown a similar rate of *decrease*. What accounts for the apparent reduction, they argue, is that a national or regional screening programme will only ever be introduced after an exceptional period of SCD incidence and thus rates are highly likely to reduce regardless of the efficacy of intervention.[1]

Despite such criticism, the Veneto study's unique features (prospective design, sample size and follow-up duration) enable it to centrally inform the current ESC screening guidelines. However such a large sample is ultimately restricted to data generated through screening programmes themselves.

Consequently, those who have been involved in the introduction of cardiac screening have more extensive data sets than their opponents which, in turn, advantages them in subsequent debates about wider implementation. Indeed ESC statements on cardiac screening in sport share the problematic features of concussion consensus statements, being similarly driven by a particularly influential group and being variously resisted but often ineffectually (e.g. from Denmark and Norway, Müller 2012). Once screening has been introduced, its advocates and practitioners perform work that perpetuates such programmes and thus consolidates if not advances the medicalization of sport.

Conclusion

If the rationale for the implementation of cardiac screening in sport is relatively weak, and the process creates rather than resolves problems for its athlete subjects, why does it exist? Athletes' compliance with cardiac screening stems in part from the fact that medical intervention is relatively commonplace in elite sport, either through routine physiological testing of performance, or the various mandatory screening programmes discussed in the introduction to this chapter. However, an understanding of the existence and persistence of cardiac screening in sport relies on an appreciation of the broader social and political dimensions of this form of medical surveillance. The introduction of screening serves the interests of (particular) members of the medical community and the nature of the screening system conspires to perpetuate its implementation.

Given that cardiac conditions do not represent a health risk to others, the tolerance of two otherwise exceptional and ethically problematic regulations (Anderson *et al.* 2012) – mandatory testing, prohibition from competitive sport – requires explanation. The perspectives of sports cardiologists provide part of the answer. Some note that, 'the cardiac arrest of a professional sportsman, who represents the essence of physical performance, has a profound psychological impact in the community' (Menafoglio *et al.* 2013: 11). Others claim that 'the devastating impact of even infrequent fatal events in the young athletic population justifies appropriate restriction from competition' (Corrado *et al.* 2011: 941; see also Anderson *et al.* 2012). While these comments accurately reflect broader social responses to SCD in sport they do not explain *why* such events have so much impact. The answer lies in the unquestioning commitment to the sport–health ideology.

Specifically, the sport–health ideology, again, leads sports to be treated as homogeneous throughout this literature. For while intensity of activity is identified as a contributory factor in SCD, in contrast to the sports injury data, the relative costs and benefits of sports-specific manifestations are rarely explored. To highlight specific sports as problematic (e.g. football) or recommend restricted participation (e.g. on the basis of differential risk for males and females) would, of course, expose flaws in the sport–health ideology by identifying more and less healthy sports and/or populations for which sports participation may be more and less harmful. It is for this reason that cardiac screening is focused on the young, who physical embody the sport–health ideology, rather than the middle-aged who are statistically at greater risk of cardiac death while playing sport. Screening as an aspect of the medicalization of sport is fundamentally enabled by, indeed might only be sustainable due to, the sport–health ideology. Cardiac screening and the sport–health ideology are therefore mutually supporting.

Note

1 This research is not without limitations. The observational and retrospective gauging of mortality rates from newspaper content analysis is less reliable than more 'objective' and prospective methods, the focus solely on competitive athletes is limiting, and the authors' claim that the newsworthiness of such incidents has remained constant is unconvincing (see Maron *et al.* 2003). However, emergency care and the prevalence of defibrillators have improved over this time, making death through cardiac arrest less frequent.

Chapter 11

Conclusion

The medicalization of sport?

In 1899 Thorstein Veblen published *The Theory of the Leisure Class* (Veblen 1899). A commentary on the consequences of capitalism as manifest in late-nineteenth century America, Veblen noted that wealthy industrialists developed lifestyles largely modelled on how they imagined previous historical elites had spent their leisure. The conspicuous consumption of non-productive time helped distance this group from the work-like activities of the masses and was taken as evidence of wealth and power. Sport in particular was envisioned as a noble activity and thus bolstered the elite's social status.

For the majority of the population, however, the essential physicality of daily life meant that sport and exercise were largely confined to brief and infrequent leisure time, especially during public holidays. There was, it should be noted, a small section of society for whom sport had become a form of employment, but on the whole participation was more closely linked to notions of belonging than distinction, and the primordial motivation stemmed from the quest for exciting significance (Elias and Dunning 1986). Sport was one of the few spheres of social life in which relatively high degrees of emotional spontaneity were afforded relatively high degrees of tolerance. For both elites and non-elites sports participation was highly gendered. It was an activity strongly contoured by age; normal for children, acceptable for young adults, unusual for their elders.

This pattern of sport participation relates to a time when the medicalization of sport was in its infancy. The primary health benefits of participation were perceived to be in relation to building character rather than shaping one's body, extending one's life or managing illness. Healthcare provision for the emerging class of sports professionals was rudimentary and frequently para-medical if not anti- or non-medical. When people became injured through sport they simply ceased to take part. This was assumed to be the natural life course.

As demonstrated throughout this book, the contemporary landscape of sport, medicine and health is clearly rather different. In most countries, and indeed a growing number, sports medicine is recognized as a distinct specialism, available to many competitive athletes and, to a greater or lesser degree, the public. Across the planet governments are instigating policies to facilitate/encourage/cajole citizens to become more physically active and, in so doing, they invariably conflate a whole range of everyday activities with both exercise and sport. A smaller but still significant and growing number of countries further regulate their populations through pre-participation screening. National and international governing bodies include an increasing array of medical issues within their ever-expanding bureaucratic regulations, defining such things as minimum levels of healthcare provision for competitive athletes and providing protocols for the management of particular conditions across their respective sports. Elite sports organizations continually seek to gain a competitive advantage by investing in the 'team behind the team'. Such is the ubiquity of the sport-medicine-health nexus that the media is replete with stories that illustrate their intersection, ranging from the innovation and organization of elite sport healthcare to 'new' scientific discoveries of the beneficial impact of exercise on the human condition. The reach of these ideas is such that significant proportions of the population structure their lives and identities around sport and exercise. At the very least, people do not fundamentally question the sport–health ideology, even if they do not feel guilty at their non-compliance.

Without doubt, this medicalization process was primarily instigated in relation to elite sport and the pursuit of competitive success. As Hoberman (1992) has amply demonstrated, physiology came to serve sports as the pursuit of performance heightened demand for scientific knowledge of the body. Yet these instances were numerically limited, culturally contested and thus, as a consequence, not as coherent and rational as has previously been proposed. Just as sport remained relatively autonomous of broader commercial developments in retaining the hegemony of amateurism, so it did when the requirements for 'fair play' necessitated a greater engagement with medicine over, e.g. drug and sex testing and when medical and scientific knowledge of training and performance came to compete against lay sporting knowledge (Carter 2009a). Here, the traditions and underlying ethos of medicine restricted its practitioners relative to less prestigious but comparably less tightly (self-)regulated professions and served to limit the contextually-evaluated worth of medicine.

Moreover, once physiologists had come to something of a consensus that vigorous levels of activity were *not* fundamentally health-harming (Heggie 2009) there was limited scope for medicine to jurisdictionally creep into the forms of sport and exercise that were seen as natural aspects of everyday life (i.e. frequent exercise during youth and increasing 'inactivity' in adulthood). Opportunities for greater medicalization primarily arose in relation to the definition of certain practices as deviant; notably injuries, in particular those incurred in contact team sports such as football and rugby and combat sports such as boxing. But medicine's limited restorative efficacy and physicians' broader ideological orientations towards the hierarchy of treatment priorities (within which SRI sat towards the bottom), represented significant barriers to the more substantive development of either medical performance-enhancement or the day-to-day service of a population conceived as fundamentally healthy. Medicine's central input was to recommend prohibition of certain practices rather than to advocate, and subsequently exert, a monopoly over treatment. The educational and class backgrounds of physicians meant that many had been deeply inculcated into the sport–health ideology, or at least the view that sport was an essential part of character building. It was therefore not surprising that concerns about the potential harm of sports participation were relatively muted. Indeed, as the case of boxing shows, medicine was as fundamental to the defence of the sport as it was to its critique.

Indeed, it seems highly likely that the relative autonomy of the elite sport sector would have continued to significantly constrain medicalization had it not been for the evocation of a broader public health remit. Within capitalist societies, medicine's ultimate dependence on state mandate restricted medicalization until a broader social worth for a specific speciality in 'sports medicine' could be demonstrated (or at least claimed). However, when a mandate did come, evident primarily as PAHP and to a lesser extent as exercise as treatment for existing conditions, the broader environmental conditions were rather less conducive to effective medicalization than they had been in the past. De-professionalization and proletarianization processes were relatively advanced and the golden age of doctoring was in clear decline (McKinley and Marceau 2002). Somewhat paradoxically, the social role of sports medicine has ultimately developed and been enabled due to bureaucratic control over state expenditure on health, the desire to rationalize and restrict the power of the medical profession, and a shift to more consumer-based, consumptive models of medicine.

The sum of these processes is that the medicalization of sport is far more apparent (or at least extensive) at the conceptual level than it is in relation to the actual practice of medical techniques and/or the engagement of patients. In many respects this is a function of the changing conceptualization of health in contemporary society (Crawford 2006) which, allied to the historic significance of the sport–health ideology, has seen a wider belief in and application of ideas that link exercise to medicinal outcomes. Pace Armstrong (1995), we might say that the medicalization of sport has been facilitated by the development of surveillance medicine, without necessarily first developing bedside or hospital forms. Constraining the more holistic medicalization of sport has been the triad of sport's relative autonomy, intra-medical conflicts which have retarded the development and restricted the jurisdictional domain of sports medicine, and state concerns to harness escalating healthcare costs. Medicine has, therefore, been more central to defining aspects of sport using its own nomenclature and paradigmatic assumptions than it has been in public intervention and implementation.

The future medicalization of sport

If the above analysis is correct, there is clearly greater potential for the medicalization of sport to expand in relation to the use of medical techniques for dealing with particular conditions and/or safeguarding participants' health. Cardiac screening and concussion are perhaps the two most developed examples, and thus central to this book. While there is considerable evidence of medicine's proactivity in this regard – evoking imperialism in places – what is perhaps most notable about these issues is that their expanded jurisdiction appears to be largely instigated by external pressure on the medical profession, especially media concerns for the health of athletes, which in turn threaten the commercial interests of sports organizations and the exposure of contradictions within the sport–health ideology more generally. In these cases, we see that somewhat self-perpetuating forces are unleashed and a degree of diffusion from elite to mass sport occurs. Not only does it seem that these external pressures will enable medicalization to develop to ever greater extents, but that such trends are largely irreversible.

An additional area in which there is considerable scope for greater medicalization is the management of sports injury within the broader population. Indeed, in some respects it is surprising that the potential social benefits of this have not been better realized already. Perhaps this is due to the forms of epidemiological data-gathering currently used and competition between branches of medicine for the 'right' to service this particular demand. But probably more important is the fact that, in this area, the social dynamics driving such developments are very different to those outlined above for, in contrast to the media publicity for some specific health issues, the most apparent driver of this form of the medicalization of sport comes from a public that appears to be increasingly intolerant of 'minor' ailments (Conrad 2007) and dissatisfied by their apparent abandonment by, or inability to access what they deem to be suitable, medicine. In line with the *health imperative*, this population experiences sport-related injury not simply as an inevitability of ageing and a sign that it is time to 'retire' from an active sporting career, but as a deeply disruptive and disturbing biographical crisis. Recognition that the more we appear to spend on healthcare the more we (as a population) report ill-health (Sen 2002), critical concerns over 'too much medicine' (Moynihan and Smith 2002) and the 'pathologization of everything' (Conrad 2007: 147) and governments' reluctance to bear the incumbent costs, act as forms of resistance. But while the numbers who might welcome this form of medicalization are significant, partly as a consequence of their heterogeneous impairments, they are disaggregated and disorganized and thus their overall influence is relatively low. It is difficult to envisage that this relatively disunited population could effectively act as a 'consumer group' seeking greater recognition for their unique and under-recognized conditions (as, for instance, has to some extent been achieved by parents of children with attention deficit hyperactivity disorder). Indeed, it seems more likely that their interests will (continue to) be serviced by smaller pockets of medical entrepreneurs who identify the commercial opportunities that such demand presents. In this respect, sports medicine may become/remain a luxury, consolidating participation trends in physical activity, the socio-economic structuring of obesity in western societies and also broader health inequalities.

In considering such potential change, it is useful to briefly sketch what an extreme scenario of sport's medicalization might look like. One can imagine a sporting landscape in which entire populations are genetically screened and then periodically medically assessed to: (a) establish personalized health risk factors which are then used to restrict the individuals' permissible range of exercise activity; and (b) generate a proscription/prescription of activities deemed medically necessary for extending life expectancy. Here, one's physical ability (matching participants for strength, speed, etc.) and nutritional and narcotic intake could be routinely monitored and used to structure when, where and against whom one might participate in sport/exercise to maximize health promotion and minimize the risk of injury. Sports trainers might cease to exist as a separate occupational entity and become largely incorporated into an increasingly diverse and stratified medical profession. Immediate and direct referral access to specialist sports medicine MDTs, with each citizen having a named physical activity healthcare advisor/provider, could either be embedded in communities as independent entities, or integrated into existing primary care provision. As with other targets of health promotion one can also envisage a scenario in which non-compliance is itself medicalized, with those who continue to resist routine participation in physical activity pathologized as in need of (different) medical intervention, much as alcoholism has become treated as a distinct form of addiction and obesity/disordered eating is increasingly viewed.

This future might entail a greater degree of convergence between elite and mass sports medicine provision than hitherto, particularly in relation to personalized medicine, pre-participation screening to channel individuals into activities for which they are genetically or physiologically predisposed and routinely medically monitoring people to guide future activity choices. But, for the select few who participate in commercial and/or nationally representative sport, medicine might also increasingly come to resemble elite occupational healthcare. Here, clinicians would be sports medicine specialists and operate a high degree of practice autonomy. As in contemporary medicine more broadly, their input would be partly shaped by consumer demand but their manifest expertise would engender significant levels of trust and confidence. Most importantly, sports administrators and coaches would exert minimal influence. Sports medicine would increasingly become an experimental rather than remedial field, leading practice innovation rather than servicing sport.

Speculation over the future extension of medicalization must be tempered with recognition of the strong countervailing forces to such developments (in sport). PAHP may be the most obvious manifestation of the medicalization of sport and may, in practice, extend medicine's jurisdictional domain to encompass hitherto untouched aspects of the life-course, but it is also fraught with contradictions that threaten to fundamentally constrain the future development of medicalization processes. Specifically, there are key questions about whether medical personnel more broadly (and not just those driving for the expansion of sports medicine) really want or are able (e.g. through possession of the relevant physical capital), to colonize what has traditionally been the jurisdictional domain of exercise professionals. Moreover, a key marker of the success of PAHP will be the reduction of illness and thus (in theory) the removal of citizens from direct medical supervision and control. PAHP, and especially data which claims the greater efficacy of exercise relative to pharmaceuticals, logically leads to the reduced influence of the medical profession and the industries that trade on its coattails (S.J. Williams *et al.* 2011). Paradoxically PAHP has been both fundamental, yet essentially antithetical, to the medicalization of sport.

Further medicalization will also be constrained by the relative expense of medicine. At a societal level these costs largely stem from the social evaluation of the professions' efficacy, but sport modalities such as physiotherapy and CAMs, which athletes seem to hold in relatively equal regard, have the obvious merit of being notably cheaper. In this regard, medicine is constrained by a prestige that relies upon distinction. The orientations of medicine compared with these other healthcare providers (including athletic therapists who, in turn, merge with elements of the fitness industry) may continue to be as inhibiting as they are enabling because status can only ever be relative, and medicine must therefore ring-fence its practices and traditions (e.g. through recourse to ethical principles) if it is to retain its identity. This, in turn must logically contribute to higher costs and subsequently restrict medicine's reach.

Other countervailing forces lay rather more outside medicine's ambit. Central to this is the influence of the sport–health ideology. As we have seen, this set of ideas (and especially where they have been threatened) has in the past been a driver of greater medicalization. However, despite an increasing array of evidence to the contrary (e.g. the incidence of concussion, the claimed necessity of cardiac screening), there is no significant body of opinion that is essentially oppositional to these beliefs. Consequently, the social valence of this ideology shows no signs of abating. As long as significant proportions of the population believe that taking part in sport activities is fundamentally good for one's health, sport-related injuries will always be somewhat counter-intuitive and the legitimacy of an associated 'sick role' (Parsons 1975) questioned. Extending the health monitoring of sports participants could of course threaten that, but as long as medicine continues to attribute 'abnormal' cases to underlying genetic causes rather than the agglomeration of lifestyle factors (perhaps including exercise) the threat will remain muted.

At the opposite end of the spectrum – the encroachment into everyday aspects of the life-course – further medicalization is restricted by two features. The first is the inherent contradictions of defining health relationally through estimations of risk as opposed to the absence or presence of 'illness' (Kreiner and Hunt 2013). It is true that this paradigm means that medicine can never fully solve the problems it explicitly seeks to resolve, for if the population's health is placed on a spectrum of life expectancy, 'abnormality' will always exist and ongoing medical intervention is always required. But equally, where the health of the population is defined in this way, the relative cultural value of particular activities (and associated body shapes) is logically reliant on the *in*ability of the entire population to comply with PAHP. Simply stated, if everyone exercised as PAHP proscribed, it would either push people into ever more extreme (and dangerous) forms of exercise or cease to be an activity of sufficient social worth to incentivize the population to exercise. The medicalization of sport, therefore, is restricted by the conceptualization of health as relative. Moreover, the conflation of health and lifestyle is inherently contradictory. The pursuit of the former is predicated on the homogenization of population outcomes while, as Veblen (1899) presciently noted, the latter entails the pursuit of heterogeneity and distinction.

The second relates to the historical continuity of motivations to take part in sport and sport-related activities. A key barrier to the acceptance of PAHP and the universal uptake of exercise is that those levels of activity that are currently believed to be most conducive to good health (i.e. minimize future health risks) are somewhat at odds with those activities to which populations are attracted. It is important in this context to re-invoke the notion of the quest for exciting significance (see Chapter 1). Simply stated, regular, gentle, rhythmic and moderate physical exercise is fundamentally different to the kind of emotional stimulation which, according to the theory of the quest for excitement (Elias and Dunning 1986), provides a central motivation to our pursuit of sport and leisure activities. This theory of the social significance of sport in modern societies remains highly applicable to current leisure trends. The growth of adventurous and lifestyle activities (Atkinson 2013), new forms of combat sports such as mixed martial arts, which frequently entail the evocation of high degrees of risk (Sanchez-Garcia and Malcolm 2010) and the propensity for more extreme degrees of endurance sports including military-inspired 'boot camp' training and Iron Man events (Atkinson 2008), suggest an ongoing or growing quest for non-routine experiences. To return again to ideas evoked in Chapter 1 – the phenomenal popularity of urban marathon running – there were an estimated 541,000 completed marathons in the USA in 2014. Not only were numbers far lower in 1980 (an estimated 140,000 completed marathons) but the activity was largely confined to young men (74% under 40, 10% women). Now, completing a marathon is a less exceptional achievement. It is no longer any great demonstration of masculinity (Smith 1998) as the gender gap has narrowed (with a male-to-female ratio of participants of 53:47) and it has become evidently attainable for older populations, with 47% of completions in 2014 by those over 40 (RunningUSA 2014). The search for exciting significance inevitably encourages people into activities that entail relatively high degrees of risk (compared with contemporary social norms, if not historically-speaking). Such activities may be highly visible contemporary spectacles of health (Nettleton and Hardey 2006) but, and highly ironically in light of the ubiquity of the sport–health ideology, the popularity of such activities is exactly because they offer something that is not entirely and inevitably health-promoting. The medicalization of sport, maximizing its health-promoting and minimizing its health-harming features, may be restricted by the limitations of political and medical understanding of participants' motives. This may be one area of social life where medicalization does not lead to a de-skilling of the population who will remain resolute in pursuing activities that engender a broader emotional stimulation.

The future study of sport, medicine and health

In drawing to a conclusion, it is important to consider what the examination of the interdependence of sport, medicine and health tells us about the broader concept of medicalization, the sociological study of health and illness more generally and the study of sport per se. Through focusing on a specific sphere of social life, one gets a particularly clear illustration of the complex and multi-level character of the broader medicalization process. This is evident, for example, in the radical differences between medicalization as manifest in PAHP and sports medicine as a form of occupational healthcare. Further, it is evident that the dynamics of medicalization are varied, sometimes with a medical profession that is pro-active and imperialistic (e.g. in relation to concussion and cardiac screening) and sometimes reluctant to extend its social influence through attempts to solve the problems of sports organizations. We can see that medicalization is complicated by the divisions inherent to a medical profession which: (a) is called upon

to take an explicit but somewhat subjective stance on aspects of contemporary living (e.g. the morality of boxing); and (b) has expanded to
encompass multiple specialities which themselves compete over jurisdictional boundaries. Such is the ubiquity and power of the broader discourse
of medicalization that it is also evident that non-medical personnel and
professions can exploit the opportunities that these developments create,
sometimes in conjunction with medicine (e.g. in MDTs), and sometimes to
medicine's disadvantage (for example, when physiotherapists contest the
position of primary care givers in the sports setting). Medicalization cannot
neatly be categorized as either a force for social good or illegitimate jurisdictional advance as such processes can lead to both public benefit (e.g. the
recognition of the potential longer term harms of head injury), and public
detriment (e.g. the sense of guilt exhibited by those whose physical condition severely restricts their ability to comply with PAHP). An absence of
medicalization, or at least its relatively limited development, can lead to
the neglect of the public (e.g. the frustrated treatment demands of those
with sports injuries) and/or their enforced engagement with a commercial
healthcare sector. While a consequence of the expansion of medical control
can be seen to be the removal of individual responsibility for particular
types of behaviour (i.e. medical recognition entails the legitimization of a
sick role and revised social responsibilities) (Conrad 2007), as the evidence
reviewed here suggests, it can also lead to victim-blaming and the appropriation of guilt to the individual rather than recognition of broader social
structural constraints. From examining sport 'in the round', the way its
macro, meso and micro levels interact, we see that medicalization is not a
unilinear or inexorable process, but contested and contingent, exhibiting
intended and unintended consequences, and an 'increasingly complex inter-
play of various social actors' (Conrad 2007: 149). As Conrad (2007: 164)
concludes,

> it is hard to imagine a world in which medicalization diminishes.
> Whatever the medical and social consequences, medicalization will
> remain a dominant approach for a range of human problems. The
> questions remain: How will medicalization affect the organization of
> society, and how will we deal with the consequences?

Also evidenced through this text is a rationale for why sport-related phenomena need to be more centrally positioned in the sociological study of
medicine, health and illness. At its core, the relatively recent establishment
of sport and exercise medicine (in the UK at least), and its global growth as
a specialism, cements it as part of the broader medical landscape of the
twenty-first century. The media exposure of elite sports medicine heightens
both public demand and expectation, and concurrently the sub-discipline
has expanded from treating a relatively narrow population to a demographic

(the entire population) that fundamentally dwarfs most other areas of medicine. The centrality of physical activity to health promotion – one of the 'big four' targets of public health – gives sport and exercise medicine a social impact that cannot be ignored, and although sociology of health and illness studies have begun to incorporate 'fitness', the exclusion of a wider range of sport-related activities necessarily limits their applicability. Moreover, arguably there is growing epidemiological and qualitative research evidence indicating that SRI is the significant bio-physical and social event that (British) sport and exercise medicine sought for many years to demonstrate. The relative increase in chronic conditions, the emphasis on ongoing self-management rather than cure and perceptions of budgetary constraint suggest that physical activity is likely to become integrated into the treatments offered in a widening range of medical fields. Conversely, this specialism illustrates the dynamics of intra-medical conflicts and of powerful social institutional resistance to the development of medical jurisdictional domains. Thus, the development of sport and exercise medicine resonates with many broader trends in medicine, exemplifying what has been described as a new medical pluralism (Cant and Sharma 1999) and, through its more detailed and extensive study, promises to throw the changes evident in cognate fields into much sharper relief.

The final stages of completing this book also further convinced me – if indeed that were needed – that the sociological study of sport would benefit from a more comprehensive analysis of medical and health-related concepts and issues. Numerous examples of the medicine-health-sport nexus emerged in the British media in the final weeks of preparing this manuscript, which not only delayed completion, but reinforced the sense that the processes this text explores are essentially incipient. These included: the NFL's admission of a link between playing American football and CTE; calls from a number of academics to ban tackling in school's rugby due to the potential injury risk and the incidence of concussion in particular; the sudden, enforced retirement of an international cricketer – James Taylor – due to the discovery of an underlying cardiac problem; calls for cardiac first aid to be incorporated into the physical education curriculum in schools; the post-fight coma of boxer Nick Blackwell; the demands for the organizers of Parkrun to contribute to the cost of staging events in local council facilities; the announcement that 2012 Paralympic medallist Erraid Davies was no longer deemed sufficiently impaired to compete in the 2016 Rio Paralympics; the retrospective positive drugs tests of 31 participants in the Beijing Olympics, 14 of whom had represented Russia; and calls for the Rio Olympic games to be relocated to inhibit the spread of the Zika virus. Indeed, I am conscious that this text is not, and was never intended to be, wholly comprehensive. Issues only cursorily addressed include performance-enhancing drug use, gender and genetic testing, the medicalization of everyday exercise through emerging technologies, the sport–health consumer market, and the treatment of the public in sports medicine clinics and hospital settings. The future expansion of themes is highly likely.

Consequently, it seems reasonable to argue that sociologists of sport need to be increasingly familiar with analyses of medicine and health more broadly if they are to be able to adequately theorize developments within this domain. Sport, medicine and health are some of the most pervasive social institutions and movements of our time and their increasing interdependence seems almost inevitable. However, it is not enough to simply assume that 'sport' will rationally appropriate what it can from medical science for equally we see evidence of the relative autonomy of sport as a social institution marked by the somewhat 'irrational' (or empirically flawed) preservation of the sport–health ideology. Similarly, sociologists of sport need to engage with the PAHP agenda and provide the empirical detail to form effective critiques of a movement that can be seen to be as much the product of changes to the political economy and the social construction of knowledge in contemporary societies as they are to the growing weight of scientific evidence. The connection here is that, fundamentally, like medicine and health, sport and exercise participation are frequently 'corporeal problems of control' (Malcolm and Mansfield 2013: 409). Sport is, and conceivably will always be, something that extends beyond the pursuit of health through physical activity, but our desires for both health and physical activity are predicated on our growing awareness of our fundamental interdependence as a population, the malleability of our biological manifestation for social ends and the impact of internalized behavioural self-control on one's relative social position. The relationships between sport, medicine and health may be contradictory and highly complex, but their social significance is both considerable and growing.

Appendix

Research note

This book is the product of around 15 years of research which began in in the broad area of the sociology of sport and has increasingly ventured into sociological aspects of medicine, health and illness. As the project developed it has increasingly engaged with the literature published in sports history and the history of medicine, the works published in medical and sports medical journals and the policy documents of both sports governing bodies and public health agencies. This much should be evident from reading the main body of the text. The central purpose of this research note, however, is to chart the seven primary empirical research projects conducted along the way and, where possible, to signal the reader to extant discussions of the methodological designs of the studies that underpin this book. The studies are described in chronological order rather than the sequence in which they appear in the text. Consequently, each is identified by a letter to facilitate cross-referencing.

A.   The journey began in 1997 when my then colleague Ken Sheard and I conducted a questionnaire survey of the top 68 clubs (response rate 41%) in the English rugby union league pyramid (the Premiership, National Leagues One and Two, and the North and South Divisions of National League Three). This research explored the impact of the relatively recent phase of commercialization on the game's organizational structure, including the changing resource priorities which, in turn, encompassed implications for healthcare provision (see Malcolm *et al.* 2000).

B.   In 2000 we followed this up with a research project funded by small grants secured from the University of Leicester's Research Fund and its Social Science Faculty Research Board. The design of this research owed a great deal to our colleagues Ivan Waddington and Martin Roderick and their collaborators Graham Parker and Rav Naik who had recently completed a project on the management of injuries in English professional football (see, for example, Roderick *et al.* 2000; Waddington 2000; and Waddington *et al.* 2001; Malcolm 2013 also provides a discussion of the impact of this research on sport, academia and on the author in particular). Again the research focused on these 68 clubs with players and coaches identified from rugby union directories, and the names and contact details of the head doctor and physiotherapist obtained by telephoning each club. A two-phase method was then employed. Between September 2000 and October 2001, 42 in-depth, semi-structured interviews were conducted with seven coaches/Directors of Rugby, nine doctors (all male), 10 physiotherapists (five female and five male) and 16 players. Our selection of interviewees combined elements of convenience and random sampling, but was partly also influenced by geographical concerns and a desire to obtain as diverse a sample as possible for the broader research project. That said, the sample was biased towards respondents from the top leagues as a consequence of differing degrees of organizational coherence and cooperation from clubs and respondents. Interviews lasted between 30 and 60 minutes and took place at rugby clubs and at healthcare professionals' (other) workplaces (e.g. surgeries and offices). Interviews were recorded and transcribed in full (primarily by the two researchers). In addition to this we administered a postal questionnaire survey to provide largely quantitative data on the qualifications, work routines and motivations of club doctors and physiotherapists. Thirty-four questionnaires (50%) were returned from rugby club doctors, and 27 (39.7%) were returned from physiotherapists. Malcolm (2006a; 2006b) contains the most complete description of the research design of this project.

C.   The richness of this body of data facilitated various publications in the subsequent years (e.g. Malcolm 2006a, 2009, 2011; Malcolm and Sheard 2002), while the broader project extended though a new collaboration, this time with Andrea Scott. A proposal for a study of 'the occupational practices of sports medicine clinicians working with British Olympic athletes' was accepted and funded by the School of Sport and Exercise Sciences at Loughborough University, and Andrea began a doctoral study under my supervision in October 2006. The target sample consisted of members of the BOA Medical Committee and BOA Physiotherapy Forum, upon which sit representatives of each of the 35 Olympic sport NGBs. Again, a two-phase research method was employed. First, questionnaires were sent to gain easily quantifiable data on career biographies, motivations and work routines and which therefore also provided data that could be compared with the studies discussed above (Malcolm 2006b; Waddington *et al.* 2001). A total of 21 doctors returned questionnaires (response rate of 60%), 18 of whom volunteered to participate further in the study and provided contact details. While attempts were made to interview all of them, 14 interviews (11 male, three female) were ultimately conducted by Andrea. Additionally, of the 20 (57%) physiotherapists who returned questionnaires, 16 volunteered to be interviewed, of whom it proved possible to arrange interviews with 14 (five male, nine female). Scott (2010) provides the most detailed accounts of the method employed in this project, although shorter descriptions appear in Malcolm and Scott (2011) and Scott and Malcolm (2015).

Subsequently the empirical research became more concentrated and increasingly focused towards the production of this book. In 2013, four discrete but concurrent projects which would come to inform the broader research programme began.

D.   First, in collaboration Andrea Scott (again) and former colleague Ivan Waddington, and supported with a grant from the Chichester University Research Facilitation Fund, we sought to examine changes to the medical provision in English professional football since Waddington *et al.*'s (2001) early study. In January 2014 questionnaires were sent to named doctors (identified via websites or by telephoning clubs) at each of the 92 clubs in the top four English football leagues. Questionnaires again explored the demographics, career backgrounds, working practices, appointment procedures and contractual basis of club doctors' roles. Thirty-three questionnaires were returned (response rates of 35.8%). Respondents were relatively evenly spread across the leagues and all were male. Developing a successful feature of the design of the earlier rugby study, a parallel questionnaire was sent to a named physiotherapist at each of the 92 clubs. Forty-two questionnaires were returned (response rate of 45.6%); all but one respondent was male. Respondents were again drawn from across the leagues although there was a notable difference between responses from League 1 (the highest response rate, 38.1%) and League 2 (the lowest, 14.3%).

Both doctors and physiotherapists were invited to provide contact details if they were interested in taking part in a subsequent interview, and ultimately it proved possible for the three of us to meet with eight doctors and 14 physiotherapists. Each was interviewed for between 30 and 60 minutes and the audio recordings were professionally transcribed. The interview schedules sought to elaborate on the biographical details already provided but particularly look at issues related to contested RTP decisions, ethical dilemmas such as maintaining patient confidentiality and the specific issues related to concussion management and cardiac screening.

E.   Concurrently I was engaged in a Department of Health funded project entitled, The Physical Activity and Respiratory Health (PhARaoH) Study. This was a large multidisciplinary and mixed method research design, led by Loughborough colleagues Lauren Sherar and Myra Nimmo and including both academic (Stuart Biddle, Dale Esliger, Andrew Kingsnorth, Mark Orme) and clinical collaborators (Mike Morgan, Sally Singh and Mike Steiner). In total, 436 adults completed a range of demographic, life history and psychological questionnaire surveys, underwent a range of physiological testing, and had their physical activity and time sedentary assessed via an accelerometer.

As the lead qualitative researcher I assembled a sub-sample of participants who had been diagnosed with COPD to participate in a one-on-one semi-structured interview in which they discussed their biography as a COPD patient, the impact of COPD on daily living, their history of, current involvement in, and barriers to physical activity and exercise. Initially, participants (from a pool of 139 COPD patients in the broader study) were contacted at random but subsequently selection became more purposive to ensure that the sub-sample contained patients exhibiting a spectrum of illness symptoms (defined by lung function and patient-reported severity; two measures that were frequently discordant). Of 34 contacted, eight failed to respond to telephone calls/answerphone messages or subsequently declined to be interviewed. In total, 26 interviews were conducted by myself (19) and Hilda Parker (seven), a research nurse trained in qualitative research methods whom I inducted into the aims and design of the study. Interviews lasting between 30 and 55 minutes were conducted in participants' homes, hospital and university facilities, or in a convenient place nominated by the participant (e.g. a supermarket cafe). Data saturation was thought to have been achieved after 23 interviews but a further three interviews were conducted, which confirmed that no new data themes were emerging. All interviews were digitally recorded and professionally transcribed as soon as possible after the interview concluded.

F.   A third study, this time funded by the Wellcome Trust, was conducted in early 2014. Again, in collaboration with a research associate, Emma Pullen, semi-structured interviews were conducted with 20 participants recruited by placing study details on the Facebook pages or noticeboards of local sports clubs or by attending training sessions. Using random and purposive sampling techniques male and female (9:11) adult participants (ages 20–56) were recruited from a range of sport and/or exercise activities. The sample exhibited a middle-class bias with many possessing higher education qualifications. Certain activities (football, tennis, and gym use) were notable absences due to a lack of co-operation from commercial gyms and some volunteer sport clubs. Interviews took place at mutually convenient locations (e.g. participants' homes, coffee shops) and lasted 20–120 minutes. They were audio recorded to provide a professionally transcribed written (verbatim) record for analysis.

G.   Finally, in March 2014, self-funded interview-based research was conducted with five 18-year-old academy players at an English Championship football club. A mutual friend provided a contact to the academy physiotherapist who facilitated a series of interviews at the training ground. Interviews lasted up to 25 minutes and included reflections on the experience and process of cardiac screening, knowledge of the background to screening and the actual and potential impact of test results on individuals. Again the recordings were transcribed (some by myself, others professionally) as soon as was practicable.

Thus, in total, the book as a whole is informed by data gathered through four questionnaire surveys and 140 interviews. While a text like this is designed to be greater than the sum of its parts, the following relationship between Chapters and projects may be useful:

Chapter 5 is largely informed by data derived from project F;
Chapter 6 from project E;
Chapters 7 and 8 from projects A–D;
Chapter 9 from projects B and D; and
Chapter 10 from projects D and G.

As should be evident from the above, very little of this would have been possible without the cooperation of my various research collaborators and I am deeply grateful to them for both the formative and enjoyable experience of conducting these projects. The views in this text are, of course, all mine and any errors attributable solely to me.

References

Abbott, A. (1988) *The System of Professions: An Essay in the Division of Expert Labour*. Chicago: University of Chicago Press.

Abbott World Marathon Majors (2015) 'Virgin Money London Marathon', www.worldmarathonmajors.com/races/london/about/. Accessed 10 January 2016.

Abernathy, L., McNally, O., MacAuley, D. and O'Neil, S. (2002) 'Sports medicine and the accident and emergency medicine specialist', *Emergency Medicine*, 40: 566.

AC Milan (2016) 'What is Milanlab?', www.acmilan.com/en/club/milan_lab. Accessed 29 March 2016.

ACSM (1990) 'Position stand: the recommended quantity and quality of exercise for developing and maintaining cardiorespiratory and muscular fitness in health adults', *Medicine and Science in Sports and Exercise*, 22: 265–274.

Adamson, C. (1997) 'Existential and clinical uncertainty in the medical encounter: an idiographic account of an illness trajectory defined by Inflammatory Bowel Disease and Avascular Necrosis', *Sociology of Health and Illness*, 19: 133–159.

Allen, D. (1997) 'The nursing-medical boundary: a negotiated order?' *Sociology of Health & Illness*, 19(4): 498–520.

Allen-Collinson, J. (2005) 'Emotions, interaction and the injured sporting body', *International Review for the Sociology of Sport*, 40(2): 221–240.

Allender, S., Foster, C., Scarborough, P. and Rayner, M. (2007) 'The burden of physical activity-related ill health in the UK', *Journal of Epidemiological Community Health*, 61: 344–348.

AMRC (2015) *Exercise: The Miracle Cure and the Role of the Doctor in Promoting it*. London: Academy of Medical Royal Colleges.

Andermann, A., Blancquaert, I., Beauchamp, S. and Déry, V. (2008) 'Revisiting Wilson and Jungner in the genomic age: a review of screening criteria over the past 40 years', *Bulletin of the World Health Organisation*, 86(4): 317–319.

Anderson, L. (2011) 'Bloodgate: were the punishments fair?', *British Journal of Sports Medicine*, 45: 948–949.

Anderson, L. and Gerrard, D.F. (2005) 'Ethical issues concerning New Zealand sports doctors', *Journal of Medical Ethics*, 31: 88–92.

Anderson, L. and Jackson, S. (2012) 'Competing loyalties in sports medicine: threats to medical professionalism in elite commercial sport', *International Review of the Sociology of Sport*, 48(2): 238–256.

Anderson, E. and Kian, E. (2012) 'Examining media contestation of masculinity and head trauma in the National Football League', *Men and Masculinities*, 15(2): 152–173.

Anderson, L., Exeter, D. and Bowyer, L. (2012) 'Sudden cardiac death: mandatory exclusion of athletes at risk is a step too far', *British Journal of Sports Medicine*, 46: 331–334.

Andrew, N.E, Wolfe, R., Cameron, P., Richardson, M., Page, R., Bucknill, A. and Gabbe, B. (2014) 'The impact of sport and active recreation injuries on physical activity levels at 12 months post-injury', *Scandinavian Journal of Medicine and Science in Sports*, 24: 377–385.

Andrews, D. (2008) 'Kinesiology's *inconvenient truth* and the physical cultural studies imperative', *Quest*, 60(1): 45–62.

APA (2011) 'Physiotherapy in Australia', www.physiotherapy.asn.au/index.php/careers/overview. Accessed 16 June 2013.

APCPA (2014) *Tackling Physical Inactivity – A Coordinated Approach*. London: All-Party Commission on Physical Activity.

Armstrong, D. (1995) 'The rise of surveillance medicine', *Sociology of Health and Illness*, 17(3): 393–404.

Armstrong, N. (2005) 'Resistance through risk: women and cervical cancer screening', *Health, Risk and Society*, 7(2): 161–176.

Armstrong, N. and Eborall, H. (2012) 'The sociology of medical screening: past, present and future', *Sociology of Health and Illness*, 34(2): 161–176.

Aronowitz, R. (2009) 'The converged experience of risk and disease', *The Milbank Quarterly*, 87(2): 417–442.

Associated Press (2013) 'NFL, ex-players agree to $765M settlement in concussions suit', NFL.Com, 29 August 2013, www.nfl.com/news/story/0ap1000000235494/article/nfl-explayers-agree-to-765m-settlement-in-concussions-suit. Accessed 9 February 2016.

Atkinson, M. (2008) 'Triathlon, suffering and exciting significance', *Leisure Studies*, 27(2): 165–180.

Atkinson, M. (2013) 'Norbert Elias: the quest for excitement in parkour', in E. Pike and S. Beames (eds), *Outdoor Activities and Social Theory*. London: Routledge.

Baarts, C. and Pederson, I. (2009) 'Derivative benefits: exploring the body through complementary and alternative medicine', *Sociology of Health and Illness*, 31(5): 719–733.

Baarveld, F., Visser, C.A., Kollen, B.J. and Backx, F.J.G. (2011) 'Sports injuries in primary health care', *Family Practice*, 28: 29–33.

Bailey, P. (2004) 'The dyspnea-anxiety-dsypnea cycle – COPD patients' stories of breathlessness: "It's scary when you can't breathe"', *Qualitative Health Research*, 14: 760–778.

Barclay, J. (1994) *In Good Hands: The History of the Chartered Society of Physiotherapy, 1894–1994*. Oxford: Butterworth Heinemann.

Batt, M. and Cullen, M. (2005) 'Sport and exercise medicine in the United Kingdom comes of age', *British Journal of Sports Medicine*, 39: 250–251.

Batt, M. and Macleod, D.A. (1997) 'The coming of age of sports medicine', *British Medical Journal*, 314: 621.

Baum, F. and Fisher, M. (2014) 'Why behavioural health promotion endures despite its failure to reduce health inequalities', *Sociology of Health and Illness*, 36(2): 213–225.

Bauman, Z. (2000) *Liquid Modernity*. Cambridge: Polity Press.

BBC (2012) 'Fabrice Muamba collapse could lead to more heart screenings', 22 March, www.bbc.co.uk/sport/0/football/17481846.

BBC (2014) 'RideLondon cyclist Kris Cook dies after bike ride collapse', 11 August 2014, www.bbc.co.uk/news/uk-england-28742179. Accessed 10 May 2016.

BBC (2015a) 'Jose Mourinho stands by criticism of Eva Carneiro and Jon Fearn', 14 August 2015, www.bbc.co.uk/sport/0/football/33931547. Accessed 29 March 2016.

BBC (2015b) 'Concussion: Saracens trial new impact-measuring device', 4 January 2015, www.bbc.co.uk/sport/rugby-union/30671380. Accessed 23 March 2016.

BBC (2015c) 'Dutee Chand: I lost all my honour in landmark gender case', 28 July 2015, www.bbc.co.uk/sport/athletics/33690274. Accessed 14 April 2016.

BBC (2015d) 'Tim Nicot: second Belgian footballer dies of cardiac arrest', 11 May 2015, www.bbc.co.uk/sport/football/32687608. Accessed 14 April 2016.

BBC (2016) 'Patrick Ekeng: Dinamo Bucharest and Cameroon midfielder dies after collapse', 7 May 2016, www.bbc.co.uk/sport/football/36234022. Accessed 10 May 2016.

Beamish, R. and Ritchie, I. (2006) *Fastest, Highest, Strongest: A Critique of High Performance Sport*. London: Routledge.

Beaumont (2012) 'Doctor selected for US Olympic Medical Staff', www.beaumont. edu/doctor-selected-us-olympic-medical-staff-summer-games-2012. Accessed 6 July 2013.

Bedford, P.J. and MacAuley, D.C. (1984) 'Attendances at a causality department for sport related injuries', *British Journal of Sports Medicine*, 18: 116–121.

Bercovitz, K. (2000) 'A critical analysis of Canada's "Active Living": science or politics?', *Critical Public Health*, 10(1): 19–39.

Bernstein, J., Perlis, C. and Bartolozzi, A.R. (2004) 'Normative ethics in sports medicine', *Clinical Orthopaedic Related Research*, 420: 309–318.

Berryman, J. (2010) 'Exercise is medicine: a historical perspective', *Current Sports Medicine Reports*, 9(4): 1–7.

Berryman, J. (2012) 'The role of physiology and cardiology in the founding and early years of the American College of Sports Medicine', in D. Malcolm and P. Safai (eds), *The Social Organization of Sports Medicine: Critical Socio-Cultural Perspectives*. New York: Routledge, 25–53.

BHF (2013) *Policy Statement: Cardiac Screening for Professional Athletes*. British Heart Foundation, www.bhf.org.uk/publications/policy-documents/screening-of-athletes, 14 April 2016.

Bille, K., Figueiras, D., Schamasch, P., Kappenberger, L., Brenner, J.I., Meijboom, F.J. and Meijboom, E.J. (2006) 'Sudden cardiac death in athletes: the Lausanne recommendations', *European Journal of Cardiovascular Prevention and Rehabilitation*, 13: 859–875.

Bloyce, D. and Smith, A. (2009) *Sport Policy and Development: An Introduction*. London: Taylor and Francis.

BMA (1996) *Sport and Exercise Medicine: Policy and Provision*. London: British Medical Association.

BOA (2006) *BOA Register of Chartered Physiotherapists in Elite Sport: Criteria and Procedures*. London: British Olympic Association.

Boeckxstaens, P., Deregt, M., Vandesype, P., Willems, S., Brusselle, G. and Sutter,

A.D (2012) 'Chronic obstructive pulmonary disease and comorbidities through the eyes of the patient', *Chronic Respiratory Disease*, 9(3): 183–191.

Borjesson, M. and Drezner, J. (2012) 'Cardiac screening: time to move forward!' *British Journal of Sports Medicine*, 46(s1): i4–i6.

Bourdieu, P. and Wacquant, L. (1992) *An Invitation to Reflexive Sociology*. Cambridge: Polity Press.

Boyce, S.H. (2001) 'The football club doctor system', *British Journal of Sports Medicine*, 35: 281.

Boyce, S.H. and Quigley, M.A. (2004) 'Review of sports injuries presenting to an accident and emergency department', *Emergency Medical Journal*, 21: 704–706.

NFL Head, Neck and Spine Committee and Bradley, B. (2013) 'NFL's 2013 protocol for players with concussions', NFL.Com, 1 October 2013, www.nfl.com/news/story/0ap2000000253716/article/nfls-2013-protocol-for-players-with-concussions. Accessed 23 March 2016.

Brenton, J. and Elliot, S. (2014) 'Undoing gender? The case of complementary and alternative medicine', *Sociology of Health and Illness*, 36(1): 91–107.

Brewin, J. (2011) 'The science behind victory', www.espnfc.com/story/937778/john-brewin-the-science-behind-victory-at-ac-milan. Accessed 6 October 2014.

Britten, N. (2002) 'Jeff Astle killed by heading ball', *Daily Telegraph*, 12 November 2002. www.telegraph.co.uk/news/uknews/1412908/Jeff-Astle-killed-by-heading-ball-coroner-rules.html. Accessed 23 March 2016.

Broglio, S., Vagnozzi, R., Sabin, M., Signoretti, S., Tavazzi, B. and Lazzarino, G. (2010) 'Concussion occurrence and knowledge in Italian football (soccer)', *Journal of Sports Science and Medicine*, 9: 418–430.

Bundon, A. and Clarke, L. (2014) ' "Keeping us from breaking": elite athletes' access to and use of complementary and alternative medicine', *Qualitative Research in Sport, Exercise and Health*, 121–138.

Burt, C.W. and Overpeck, M.D. (2001) 'Emergency visits for sports-related injuries', *Annals of Emergency Medicine*, 37(3): 301–308.

Bury, M. (1982) 'Chronic illness as biographical disruption', *Sociology of Health and Illness*, 4(2): 167–182.

Bury, M. (2001) 'Illness narratives: fact or fiction?', *Sociology of Health and Illness*, 23(3): 263–285.

Bury, T. and Stokes, E. (2013) 'A global view of direct access and patient self-referral to physical therapy: implications for the profession', *Physical Therapy*, 80: 28–43.

Bushby, H., Williams, G. and Rogers, A. (1997) 'Bodies of knowledge: lay biomedical understandings of musculoskeletal disorders', *Sociology of Health and Illness*, 19(19B): 79–99.

Cant, S. and Sharma, U. (1999) *A New Medical Pluralism? Alternative Medicine, Doctors, Patients and the State*. London: UCL Press.

Carmel, S. (2006) 'Boundaries obscured and boundaries reinforced: incorporation as a strategy of occupational enhancement for intensive care', *Sociology of Health & Illness*, 28(2): 154–177.

Caron, J., Bloom, G., Johnston, K. and Sabiston, C. (2013) 'Effects of multiple concussions on retired National Hockey League players', *Journal of Sport and Exercise Psychology*, 35: 168–179.

Carricaburu, D. and Pierret, J. (1995) 'From biographical disruption to biographical reinforcement: the case of HIV-positive men', *Sociology of Health and Illness*, 17(1): 65–88.

Carter, N. (2007) 'Metatarsals and magic sponges: English football and the development of sports medicine', *Journal of Sport History*, 31(1): 53–73.

Carter, N. (2009a) 'The rise and fall of the magic sponge: football trainers and the persistence of popular medicine', *Social History of Medicine*, 23(2): 261–279.

Carter, N. (2009b) 'Mixing business with leisure? The football club doctor, sports medicine and the voluntary tradition', *Sport in History*, 29(1): 69–91.

Carter, N. (2012a) *Medicine, Sport and the Body: A Historical Perspective.* London: Bloomsbury.

Carter, N. (2012b) 'From voluntarism to specialization: sports medicine and the British Association of Sport and Medicine', in D. Malcolm and P. Safai (eds) *The Social Organization of Sports Medicine: Critical Socio-Cultural Perspectives.* New York: Routledge, 54–76.

Cassell, E.P., Finch, C.F. and Stathakis, V.Z. (2003) 'Epidemiology of medically treated sport and active recreation injuries in the Latrobe Valley, Victoria, Australia', *British Journal of Sports Medicine*, 37: 405–409.

Casson, I. Viano, D., Powell, J. and Pellman, E. (2010) 'Twelve years of National Football League concussion data', *Sport Health*, 2(6): 471–483.

Cavanaugh, S. and Sykes, H. (2006) 'Transsexual bodies at the Olympics: the International Olympic Committee's policy on transsexual athletes at the 2004 Athens summer games', *Body and Society*, 12(3): 75–102.

Chandra, N., Papadakis, M. and Sharma, S. (2012) 'Cardiac adaptation in athletes of black ethnicity: differentiating pathology from physiology', *Heart*, doi:10.1136/heartjnl-2012–301798.

Clarke, L. (2015) 'Explaining NFL's concussion protocol, the five-step map for RGIII's return', *Washington Post*, 29 August 2015, www.washingtonpost.com/news/football-insider/wp/2015/08/29/explaining-nfl-concussion-protocol-the-five-step-map-for-rgiiis-return/. Accessed 23 March 2016.

Coghlan, A. (2012) 'Should athletes be screened for heart problems?', *New Scientist*, March 21, www.newscientist.com/article/dn21615-should-athletes-be-screened-for-heart-problems.html.

Conrad, P. (1987) 'The experience of illness: recent and new directions', in J. Roth and P. Conrad (eds), *Research in the Sociology of Healthcare: A Research Annual, Vol. 6. The Experience and Management of Chronic Illness.* Greenwich: Jai Press, 1–31.

Conrad, P. (1992) 'Medicalization and social control', *Annual Review of Sociology*, 18: 209–232.

Conrad, P. (2007) *The Medicalization of Society: On the Transformation of Human Conditions into Treatable Disorders.* London: Johns Hopkins University Press.

Cooper, R., Bissell, P., Ward, P., Murphy, E., Anderson, C., Avery, T., James, V., Lymn, J., Guillaume, L., Hutchinson, A. and Ratcliffe, J. (2011) 'Further challenges to medical dominance? The case of nurse and pharmacist supplementary prescribing', *Health*, 16(2): 115–133.

Corrado, D., Pelliccia, A., Bjornstad, H., Vanhees, L., Biffi, A., Borjesson, M., Panhuyzen-Goedkoop, N., Deligiannis, A., Solberg, E., Dugmore, D., Mellwig, K.P., Assanelli, D., Delise, P., van-Buuren, F., Anastasakis, A., Heidbuchel, H.,

Hoffmann, E., Fagard, R., Priori, S.G., Basso, C., Arbustini, E., Blomstrom-Lundqvist, C., McKenna, W.J. and Thiene, G. (2005) 'Cardiovascular pre-participation screening of young competitive athletes for prevention of sudden death: proposal for a common European protocol', *European Heart Journal*, 26: 516–524.

Corrado, D., Schmied, C., Basso, C., Borjesson, M., Schiavon, M., Pellica, A., Vanhees, L. and Thiene, G. (2011) 'Risk of sports: do we need a pre-participation screening for competitive and leisure athletes?' *European Heart Journal*, 32: 934–944.

Craton, N. and Leslie, O. (2014) 'Time to re-think the Zurich guidelines? A critique on the consensus statement on concussion in sport, held in Zurich, November 2012', *Clinical Journal of Sports Medicine*, 24(2): 93–95.

Crawford, C. (2016) 'Essendon players' "lack of curiosity" condemned at Court of Arbitration for Sport', www.heraldsun.com.au/news/essendon-players-lack-of-curiosity-condemned-at-court-of-arbitration-for-sport/news-story/1955e99296ef c6e8c4c7d74cd56f73dc. Accessed 29 March 2016.

Crawford, R. (1980) 'Healthism and the medicalization of everyday life', *International Journal of Health Services*, 10(3): 365–388.

Crawford, R. (2006) 'Health as a meaningful social practice', *Health*, 10(4): 401–420.

Cronin, M. (2007) 'Not taking the medicine: sportsmen and doctors in late nineteenth century Britain', *Journal of Sport History*, 34(1): 23–36.

Crossley, N. (2006) 'In the gym: motives, meaning and moral careers', *Body and Society*, 12(3): 23–50.

CSP (2008) *Charting the Future of Physiotherapy*. London: Chartered Society of Physiotherapy.

Daly, J. (1989) 'Innocent murmurs: echocardiography and the diagnosis of cardiac normality', *Sociology of Health and Illness*, 11(2): 99–116.

Dashper, K. (2013) 'Getting better: an autoethnographic tale of recovery from sporting injury', *Sociology of Sport Journal*, 30(3): 323–339.

Davis, J. (2006) 'How medicalization lost its way', *Society*, 43(6): 51–56.

de Loes, M. (1990) 'Medical treatment and costs of sports-related injuries in a total population', *International Journal of Sports Medicine*, 11: 66–72.

de Menezes, J. (2015) 'US Soccer ban heading the ball for children over fears of concussion and head injuries', *The Independent*, 10 November 2015, www.independent.co.uk/sport/football/news-and-comment/us-soccer-ban-heading-the-ball-for-children-over-fears-of-concussion-and-head-injuries-a6728341.html. Accessed 13 February 2016.

De Swaan, A. (1988) *In Care of the State: Health Care, Education, and Welfare in Europe and America during the Modern Era*. Oxford: Oxford University Press.

De Swaan, A. (1989) 'The reluctant imperialism of the medical profession', *Social Science and Medicine*, 28(11): 1165–1170.

Deane, S. (2014) 'Star's courageous brain-injury battle', *The New Zealand Herald*, 31 May 2014, www.nzherald.co.nz/nz/news/article.cfm?c_id=1&objectid=11264933. Accessed 29 February 2016.

Dekker, R., Groothoff, J.W., Van Der Sluis, C.K., Eisma, W.H. and Ten Duis, H.J. (2003a) 'Long term disabilities and handicaps following sports injuries: outcome after outpatient treatment', *Disability and Rehabilitation*, 25(2): 1153–1157.

Dekker, R., Van Der Sluis, C.K., Groothoff, J.W., Eisma, W.H. and Ten Duis, H.J. (2003b) 'Long term outcome of sports injuries: results after inpatient treatment', *Clinical Rehabilitation*, 17: 480–487.

Delaney, J., Al-Kahmiri, A., Drummond, R. and Correa, J. (2008) 'The effect of protective headgear on head injuries and concussions in adolescent football (soccer) players', *British Journal of Sports Medicine*, 42: 110–115.

Devitt, B.M. and McCarthy, C. (2010) ' "I am in blood Stepp'd in so far..." Ethical dilemmas and the sports team doctor', *British Journal of Sports Medicine*, 44: 175–78.

Dingwall, R. (1983) 'Introduction', in R. Dingwall, and P. Lewis (eds), *The Sociology of the Professions: Lawyers, Doctors and Others*. London: Macmillan, 1–13.

DNH (1995) *Sport – Raising the Game*. London: DNH.

DoH (2004) *At Least Five a Week: Evidence of the Impact of Physical Activity and its Relationship with Health*. London: DoH.

DoH (2007) *Tackling Obesities: Future Choices*. London: DoH.

DoH (2009a) *Be Active, be Healthy*. London: DoH.

DoH (2009b) *Let's get Moving*. London: DoH.

DoH (2011) *Start Active, Stay Active: Report on Physical Activity in the UK*. London: DoH.

Driscoll, D. (2013) Interview, PM radio programme, BBC Radio 4, 16 April 2013.

Dunn, S.R., George, M.S., Churchill, L. and Spindler, K.P. (2007) 'Ethics in sports medicine', *American Journal of Sports Medicine*, 35: 840–844.

Dunning, E. and Hughes, J. (2013) *Norbert Elias, Sociology and the Human Crisis: Interdependence, Power, Process*. Cambridge, UK: Polity.

Edwards, S. and McNamee, M. (2006) 'Why sports medicine is not medicine', *Health Care Analysis*, 14: 103–109.

Egger, G. (1991) 'Sport injuries in Australia: causes, cost and prevention', *Health Promotion Journal of Australia*, 1: 28–33.

Eime, R., Charity, M., Harvey, J., and Payne, W. (2015) 'Participation in sport and physical activity: associations with socio-economic status and geographical remoteness', *BMC Public Health*, 15: 434–437.

Elbe, A. and Overbye, M. (2013) 'Urine doping controls: the athletes' perspective', *International Journal of Sport Policy and Politics*.

Elias, N. (1974) 'The sciences: towards a theory', in R. Whitely (ed.), *Social Processes of Scientific Development*. London: Routledge & Kegan Paul, 21–42.

Elias, N. (1978) *What is Sociology?* London: Hutchison.

Elias, N. (1986a) 'The genesis of sport as a sociological problem', in N. Elias, and E. Dunning, *Quest for Excitement: Sport and Leisure in the Civilising Process*. Blackwell: Oxford, 126–149.

Elias, N. (1986b) 'An essay on sport and violence', N. Elias, and E. Dunning, *Quest for Excitement: Sport and Leisure in the Civilising Process*. Blackwell: Oxford, 150–174.

Elias, N. (1987) *Involvement and Detachment*. Oxford: Blackwell.

Elias, N. (2000) *The Civilizing Process: Sociogenetic and Psychogenetic Investigations* (3rd edn). Oxford: Blackwell.

Elias, N. and Dunning, E. (1986) *Quest for Excitement: Sport and Leisure in the Civilising Process*. Blackwell: Oxford.

Elias, N. and Scotson, J. (1994) *The Established and the Outsiders* (2nd edn). Sage: London.

Elston, J. and Stein, K. (2011) 'Public health implications of establishing a national programme to screen young athletes in the UK', *British Journal of Sports Medicine*, 45: 576–582.

EMJ (2008) 'Medical services at the 2012 Olympic Games and Paralympic Games: an interview with Richard Budgett', *Emergency Medicine Journal*, May Supplement. www.udel.edu/PT/PT%20Clinical%20Services/journalclub/sojc/11_12/May/EMJ-Medical%20Services%20at%202012%20Olympic%20Games.pdf. Accessed 30 March 2016.

Engebretsen, L., Soligard, T., Steffen, K., Alonso, J.M., Aubry, M., Budgett, R., Dvorak, J., Jegathesan, M., Meeuwisse, W.H., Mountjoy, M., Palmer-Green, D., Vanhegan, I. and Renström, P.A. (2013) 'Sports injuries and illnesses during the London Summer Olympic Games 2012', *British Journal of Sports Medicine*, 47(7): 407–414.

European Union (2008) *EU Physical Activity Guidelines: Recommended Policy Actions in Support of Health-enhancing Physical Activity*. http://ec.europa.eu/sport/library/policy_documents/eu-physical-activity-guidelines-2008_en.pdf. Accessed 30 March 2016.

European Union (2011) *Developing the European Dimension in Sport*. http://eur-lex.europa.eu/LexUriServ/LexUriServ.do?uri=COM:2011:0012:FIN:EN:PDF. Accessed 30 March 2016.

FA (2015) *Rules and Regulations of the Association. Season 2014–15*. London: Football Association.

Faircloth, C., Boylstein, C., Rittman, M., Young, M.E. and Gubrium, J. (2004) 'Sudden illness and biographical flow in narratives of stroke recovery', *Sociology of Health and Illness*, 26(2): 242–261.

Ferguson, D. (2013) 'Rugby players are "cheating" concussion protocols', *The Scotsman*, 27 July 2013, www.scotsman.com/sport/rugby-union/rugby-players-are-cheating-concussion-protocols-1-3017722. Accessed 29 February 2016.

FIMS (2015) www.fims.org/. Accessed 10 February 2015.

Finch, C.F. (2012) 'Getting sports injury prevention on to public health agendas – addressing the shortfalls in current information sources', *British Journal of Sports Medicine*, 46(1): 70–74.

Finch, C. and Kenihan, M. (2001) 'A profile of patients attending sports medicine clinics', *British Journal of Sports Medicine*, 35: 251–256.

Finch, C., Little, C. and Garnham, A. (2001) 'Quality of life improvements after sports injury', *Injury Control and Safety Promotion*, 8(2): 113–115.

Fox, R.C. (2000) 'Medical uncertainty revisited', in G.L. Albrecht, R. Fitzpatrick and S.C. Scrimshaw (eds), *The Handbook of Social Studies in Health and Medicine*. London: Sage, 409–425.

Fraas, M., Coughlan, G., Hart, E. and McCarthy, C. (2013) 'Concussion history and reporting rates in elite Irish rugby union players', *Physical Therapy in Sport*, http://dx.doi.org/10.1016/j.ptsp. 2013.08.002.

Frank, A. (1995) *The Wounded Storyteller: Body, Illness, and Ethics*. London: University of Chicago Press.

Freidson, E. (1970) *Profession of Medicine: A Study of the Sociology of Applied Knowledge*. New York: Dodd, Mead & Co.

Freund, P. and Martin, G. (2004) 'Walking and motoring: fitness and the social organisation of movement', *Sociology of Health and Illness*, 26(3): 273–286.

Frey, J.H. (1991) 'Social risk and the meaning of sport', *Sociology of Sport Journal*, 8: 136–145.

Fuller, C., Taylor, A. and Raferty, M. (2014) 'Epidemiology of concussion in men's elite rugby-7s (Sevens World Series) and rugby-15s (Rugby World Cup, Junior World Championship and Rugby Trophy, Pacific Nations Cup and English Premiership)', *British Journal of Sports Medicine*, Published online first, 24 February 2014, doi:10.1136/bjsports-2013-093381.

Gale, N. (2011) 'From body-talk to body-stories: body work in complementary and alternative medicine', *Sociology of Health and Illness*, 33(2): 237–251.

Gani, A. (2016) 'London Marathon runner David Seath dies after collapsing near finish line', *Guardian*, 25 April 2016, www.theguardian.com/uk-news/2016/apr/25/london-marathon-runner-capt-david-seath-dies-collapsing-near-finish-line. Accessed 10 May 2016.

Gard, M. (2010) *The End of the Obesity Epidemic*. London: Routledge.

Gard, M. and Wright, J. (2004) *The Obesity Epidemic. Science, Morality and Ideology*. London: Routledge.

Georgoulis, A.D., Kiapidou, I.S., Velogianni, L., Stergiou, N. and Boland, A. (2007) 'Herodicus, the father of sports medicine', *Knee Surgery Sports Traumatology Arthroscopy*, 15(3): 315–8.

Gilmore, S. and Sillince, J. (2014) 'Institutional theory and change: the deinstitutionalization of sports science at Club X', *Journal of Organizational Change Management*, 27(2): 314–330.

Glassner, B. (1990) 'Fit for postmodern selfhood', in H. Becker and M. McCall (eds), *Symbolic Interactionism and Cultural Studies*. Chicago: Chicago University Press.

Goudsblom, J. (1986) 'Public health and the civilizing process', *The Milbank Quarterly*, 64(2): 161–188.

Green, M. and Houlihan, B. (2005) *Elite Sport Development: Policy Learning and Political Priorities*. London: Routledge.

Guttmann, A. (1978) *From Ritual to Record: The Nature of Modern Sport*. New York: Columbia University Press.

Halfmann, D. (2011) 'Recognizing medicalization and demedicalization: discourses, practices and identities', *Health*, 16(2): 186–207.

Hamilton, B., Levine, B., Thompson, P. and Whyte, G. (2012) 'Debate: challenges in sports cardiology; US versus European approaches', *British Journal of Sports Medicine*, 46(s1): i9–i14.

Hansen, E., Walters, J. and Wood-Baker, R. (2007) 'Explaining chronic obstructive pulmonary disease (COPD): perceptions of the role played by smoking', *Sociology of Health and Illness*, 29(5): 730–749.

Hargreaves, J. (1986) *Sport, Power and Culture: A Social and Historical Analysis of Popular Sports in Britain*. Cambridge: Polity Press.

Hawkins, R. and Fuller, C. (1999) 'A prospective epidemiological study of injuries in four English professional football clubs', *British Journal of Sports Medicine*, 33: 196–203.

Heggie, V. (2008) '"Only the British appear to be making a fuss": the science of success and the myth of amateurism at the Mexico Olympiad, 1968', *Sport in History*, 28(2): 213–235.

Heggie, V. (2009) 'A century of cardiomythology: exercise and the heart c.1880–1980', *Social History of Medicine*, 23(2): 280–298.

Heggie, V. (2010a) 'Specialization without the hospital: the case of British sports medicine', *Medical History*, 54 (2010): 457–474.

Heggie, V. (2010b) 'Testing sex and gender in sports; reinventing, reimagining and reconstructing histories', *Endeavour*, 34(4): 157–163.

Heggie, V. (2011) *A History of British Sports Medicine*. Manchester, Manchester University Press.

Helm, T. (2014) 'NHS chief urges hospital staff to join gyms in anti-obesity fight', *Guardian*, 18 October 2014, www.theguardian.com/society/2014/oct/18/hospital-staff-urged-to-set-example-obesity-fight. Accessed 21 September 2015.

Heyman, B. (2010) 'Screening for health risks: a social science perspective', *Health, Risk and Society*, 12(1): 1–6.

Hillis, W.S., Stewart, K., Burns, M., Kidd, A., Maclean, J. and Macintyre, P.D. (2011) 'Preparticipation cardiovascular screening: application of an extended Italian model in Scotland', *British Journal of Sports Medicine*, 45:e2.

HM Govt and Mayor of London (2014) *Moving More, Living More. The Physical Activity Olympic and Paralympic Legacy for the Nation*. London: HM Govt and Mayor of London.

Hoberman, J. (1992) *Mortal Engines: The Science of Performance and the Dehumanization of Sport*. New York: Free Press.

Hockey, J. and Allen-Collinson, J. (2009) 'The sensorium at work: the sensory phenomenology of the working body', *The Sociological Review*, 57(2): 217–239.

Hockey, R. and Knowles, M. (2000) 'Sports injuries', *Injury Bulletin No. 59*, Queensland Injury Surveillance Unit.

Horrocks, C. and Johnson, S. (2014) 'A socially situated approach to inform health and wellbeing', *Sociology of Health and Illness*, 36(2): 175–186.

Howe, P.D. (2001) 'An ethnography of pain and injury in professional rugby union: from embryo to infant at Pontypridd RFC', *International Review for the Sociology of Sport*, 35: 289–303.

Howe, P.D. and Jones, C. (2006) 'Classification of disabled athletes: (dis)empowering the Paralympic practice community', *Sociology of Sport Journal*, 23: 29–46.

Howson, A. (1999) 'Cervical screening, compliance and moral obligation', *Sociology of Health and Illness*, 21: 401–425.

HSCIC (2014a) *Provisional Monthly Topic of Interest: Admitted Patient Care Emergency Admissions and Unplanned Accident and Emergency Attendances Caused by Road Traffic Accidents*. www.hscic.gov.uk/catalogue/PUB16284/prov-mont-hes-admi-outp-ae-April%202014%20-%20September%202014-toi-rep.pdf. Accessed 23 March 2016.

HSCIC (2014b) *Statistics on Obesity, Physical Activity and Diet: England 2014*. www.hscic.gov.uk/catalogue/PUB13648/Obes-phys-acti-diet-eng-2014-rep.pdf. Accessed 23 March 2016.

Hughes, D. (2014) 'Premier League tackling mental health', www.bbc.co.uk/news/health-29543252. Accessed 14 October 2014.

Huizenga, R. (1995) *You're Okay, It's Just a Bruise*. New York: St. Martin's Griffin.

Hutson, D. (2013) ' "Your body is your business card": bodily capital and health authority in the fitness industry', *Social Science and Medicine*, 90: 63–73.

IAAF (2012) *IAAF Medical Manual*. www.iaaf.org/about-iaaf/documents/medical. 14 April 2016.

Illich, I. (1975) *Medical Nemesis*. London: Calder & Boyers.

IOC (2003) *Statement of the Stockholm Consensus on Sex Reassignments in Sports*. www.olympic.org/documents/reports/en/en_report_905.pdf. Accessed 14 April 2016.

IRB (2008) 'Regulations relating to the game', *International Rugby Board Regulations*. www.irb.com/mm/document/lawsregs/0/reg10a4feb08_4420.pdf. Accessed Retrieved 11 March 2008.

IRB (n.d.) *World Rugby Cardiac Screening*. http://playerwelfare.worldrugby.org/?subsection=37. Accessed 14 April 2016.

James, D. (2012) 'Calls for more heart screenings simply do not add up', *Observer*, March 24, www.theguardian.com/football/blog/2012/mar/24/fabrice-muamba-heart-screenings. Accessed 14 April 2016.

Jensen, G., Gwyer, J., Shephard, K. and Hack, L. (2000) 'Expert practice in physical therapy', *Physical Therapy*, 80(1): 28–43.

Johnson, T. (1972) *Professions and Power*. London: Macmillan.

Johnson R. (2004) 'The unique ethics of sports medicine', *Clinics in Sports Medicine*, 23(2): 175–182.

Johnson, P. (2016) 'Simon Stevens: trying to steer the NHS through tumultuous times', *Guardian*, Monday 18 January, www.theguardian.com/society/2016/jan/18/simon-stevens-trying-save-nhs-from-mother-of-messes?CMP=share_btn_link.

Jonas, S. (2009) 'Introduction: what this book is about', in S. Jonas, and E. Philips (eds), *ACSM's Exercise is Medicine: A Clinician's Guide to Exercise Prescription*. Philadelphia: Lippincott, Williams and Wilkins, 1–12.

Jonas, S and Philips, E. (eds) (2009) *ACSM's Exercise is Medicine: A Clinician's Guide to Exercise Prescription*. Philadelphia: Lippincott, Williams and Wilkins.

Jones, L. and Green, J. (2006) 'Shifting discourses of professionalism: a case study of general practitioners in the United Kingdom', *Sociology of Health & Illness*, 28(7): 927–950.

Jones, R.S and Taggart, T. (1994) 'Sport related injuries attending the accident and emergency department', *British Journal of Sports Medicine*, 28(2): 110–111.

Jones, N., Weiler, R., Hutchings, K., Stride, M., Adejuwon, A., Baker, P., Larkin, J. and Chew, S. (2011) *Sport and Exercise Medicine: A Fresh Approach*. London: NHS Sport and Exercise Medicine Services.

Jordan, B. (2013) 'The clinical spectrum of sport-related traumatic brain injury', *National Review of Neurology*, 9: 222–230.

Junge, A., Engbretsen, L. and Mountjoy, M. (2009) 'Sports injuries during the summer Olympic Games 2008', *American Journal of Sports Medicine*, 37(11): 2165–2172.

Jutel, A. (2009) 'Sociology of diagnosis: a preliminary review', *Sociology of Health and Illness*, 38(2): 387–399.

Jutel, A. and Buetow, S. (2007) 'A picture of health?: unmasking the role of appearance in health', *Perspectives in Biology and Medicine*, 50(3): 421–434.

Kelleher, D., Gabe, J. and Williams, G. (1994) 'Understanding medical dominance in the modern world', in J. Gabe, D. Kelleher, and G. Williams (eds), *Challenging Medicine*. London: Routledge, xi–xxix.

Kennedy, K.W. (1990) 'The team doctor in rugby union football', in S.D.W. Payne (ed.), *Medicine, Sport and the Law*. Oxford: Blackwell, 315–323.

Kerr, R. (2012) 'Integrating scientists into the sports environment. A case study of gymnastics in New Zealand', *Journal of Sport and Social Issues*, 36(1): 3–24.

Kilminster, R. (2004) 'From distance to detachment: knowledge and self-knowledge in Elias's theory of involvement and detachment', in S. Loyal and S. Quilley (eds), *The Sociology of Norbert Elias*. Cambridge: Cambridge University Press, 25–41.

Kirkwood, G., Parekh, N., Ofori-Asenso, R. and Pollock, A. (2015) 'Concussion in youth rugby union and rugby league: a systematic review', *British Journal of Sports Medicine*, 2015;0:1–5. doi10.1136/bjsports-2014–093774 (Published online first).

Kisser, R. and Bauer, R. (2012) *The Burden of Sport Injuries in the European Union. Research Report D2h of the Project "Safety in Sports"*. Vienna: Austrian Road Safety Board.

Knill-Jones, R. (1997) 'Sports injury clinics', *British Journal of Sports Medicine*. 31: 95–96.

Kohl, H., Craig. C. and Lambert, E. (2012) 'The pandemic of physical inactivity: global action for public health', *The Lancet*, 380: 294–305.

Kotarba, J. (2001) 'Conceptualizing sports medicine as occupational health care: illustrations from professional rodeo and wrestling', *Qualitative Health Research*, 11(6): 766–779.

Kotarba, J. (2012) 'Women professional athletes' injury care: the case of women's football', in D. Malcolm and P. Safai (eds), *The Social Organization of Sports Medicine: Critical Socio-cultural Perspectives*. New York: Routledge, 107–125.

Kreiner, M. and Hunt, L. (2013) 'The pursuit of preventive care for chronic illness: turning healthy people into chronic patients', *Sociology of Health and Illness*, 36(6): 870–884.

Lancet (2012) 'Chariots of fries', *The Lancet*, 380: 9838, 188.

Larkin, G. (1983) *Occupational Monopoly and Modern Medicine*. London: Tavistock.

Larson, M.S. (1977) *The Rise of Professionalism: A Sociological Analysis*. Berkeley: University of California Press.

Leder, D. (1990) *The Absent Body*. Chicago: Chicago University Press.

Lee, C.T., Williams, P. and Hadden, W.A. (1999) 'Parachuting for charity: is it worth the money? A 5-year audit of parachute injuries in Tayside and the cost to the NHS', *Injury*, 30(4): 283–287.

Lee, I., Shiroma, E.J., Lobelo, F., Puska, P., Blair, S.N. and Katzmarzyk, P.T. (2012) 'Effect of physical inactivity on major non-communicable diseases worldwide: an analysis of burden of disease and life expectancy', *The Lancet*, 380: 219–229.

Legh-Jones, H. and Moore, S. (2012) 'Network social capital, social participation, and physical inactivity in an urban adult population', *Social Science and Medicine*, 74: 1362–1367.

Lenskyj, H. (1986) *Out of Bounds: Women, Sport and Sexuality*. Ontario: Women's Press.

Light, D. (1979) 'Uncertainty and control in professional training', *Journal of Health and Social Behavior*, 20: 310–322.

Lindqvist, G. and Hallberg, L. (2010) ' "Feelings of guilt due to self-inflicted disease": a grounded theory of suffering from chronic obstructive pulmonary disease (COPD)', *Journal of Health Psychology*, 15(3): 456–466.

Ljungqvist, A., Jenoure, P. and Engebretsen, L. (2009) *The International Olympic Committee Consensus Statement on Periodic Health Evaluation of Elite Athletes.* www.olympic.org/Documents/Reports/EN/en_report_1448.pdf.   Accessed   16 April 2016.

Locock, L., Ziebland, S. and Dumelow, C. (2009) 'Biographical disruption, abruption and repair in the context of Motor Neurone Disease', *Sociology of Health and Illness*, 31(7): 1043–1058.

LOCOG (2012) *Olympic Games Healthcare Guide.* London: LOCOG.

Lupton D. (1995) *The Imperative of Health. Public Health and the Regulated Body.* London: Sage.

Lupton, D. (1997) 'Doctors on the medical profession', *Sociology of Health & Illness*, 19(4): 480–497.

Lutfey, K. and McKinlay, J. (2009) 'What happens along the diagnostic pathway to CHD treatment? Qualitative results concerning cognitive processes', *Sociology of Health and Illness*, 31(7): 1077–1092.

MacDonald, K.M. (1995). *The Sociology of the Professions.* London: Sage.

Mackay, R. (2001) 'Club doctors and physiotherapists', *British Journal of Sports Medicine*, 35: 207.

Magalski, A., Maron, B., Main, M., McCoy, M., Florez, A., Reid, K., Epps, H., Bates, J. and Browne, J. (2008) 'Relation of race to electrocardiographic patterns in elite American football players', *Journal of the American College of Cardiology*, 51(23): 2250–2255.

Maguire, J. (1992) 'Towards a sociological theory of the emotions: a process sociological perspective', in E. Dunning and C. Rojek (eds), *Sport and Leisure in The Civilizing Process.* London: Macmillan, 96–120.

Makdissi, M., Davis, G. and McCrory, P. (2014) 'Updated guidelines for the management of sports-related concussion in general practice', *Australian Family Physician*, 43(3): 94–99.

Malcolm, D. (2006a) 'Unprofessional practice? The status and power of sports physicians', *Sociology of Sport Journal*, 23(4): 376–395.

Malcolm, D. (2006b) 'Sports medicine: a very peculiar practice? Doctors and physiotherapists in elite English rugby union', in I. Waddington, B. Skirstad and S. Loland (eds), *Pain and Injury in Sport. Social and Ethical Analysis.* London: Routledge, 165–182.

Malcolm, D. (2009) 'Medical uncertainty and clinician-athlete relations: the management of concussion injuries in rugby union', *Sociology of Sport Journal*, 26(2): 191–210.

Malcolm, D. (2011) 'Sports medicine, injured athletes and Norbert Elias's sociology of knowledge', *Sociology of Sport Journal*, 28: 284–302.

Malcolm, D. (2012) *Sport and Sociology.* London: Routledge.

Malcolm, D. (2013) 'Medical management in professional football: some reflections', in I. Waddington and A. Smith (eds), *Doing Real World Research in Sports Studies*, London: Routledge, 26–30.

Malcolm, D. (2016) 'Confidentiality in sports medicine', *Clinics in Sports Medicine*, 35: 205–215.

Malcolm, D. and Mansfield, L. (2013) 'The quest for exciting knowledge: developments in figurational sociological research on sport and leisure', *Politica & Sociedad*, 50(2): 397–419.

Malcolm, D. and Pullen, E. (forthcoming) 'Is Exercise Medicine?', in L. Mansfield, J. Piggin and M. Weed (eds), *Handbook of Physical Activity: Policy, Politics and Practice*. London: Routledge.

Malcolm, D. and Safai, P. (2012) *The Social Organization of Sports Medicine: Critical Socio-Cultural Perspectives*. New York: Routledge.

Malcolm, D. and Scott, A. (2011) 'Professional relations in elite sport healthcare: workplace responses to organisational change', *Social Science and Medicine*, 72(4): 513–520.

Malcolm, D. and Scott, A. (2014) 'Practical responses to confidentiality dilemmas in elite sport medicine', *British Journal of Sports Medicine*, 48(19): 1410–1413.

Malcolm, D. and Sheard, K. (2002) ' "Pain in the assets": the effects of commercialization and professionalization on the management of injury in English rugby union', *Sociology of Sport Journal*, 19(2): 149–169.

Malcolm, D. and Smith, A. (2015) 'Football and performance enhancing drugs', in I. Waddington, J. Hoberman and V. Moller (eds), *The Routledge Companion to Sport and Drugs*. London: Routledge, 103–114.

Malcolm, D., Sheard, K. and White, A. (2000) 'The changing structure and culture of English rugby union football', *Culture, Sport, Society*, 3(1): 63–87.

Malcolm, D., Sheard, K. and Smith, S. (2004) 'Protected research: sports medicine and rugby injuries', *Sport in Society*, 7(1): 97–110.

Mansfield, L. and Malcolm, D. (2014) 'The Olympic movement, sport and health', in J. Baker, J.-F. Thomas and P. Safai (eds), *Health and Elite Sport: Is High Performance Sport a Healthy Pursuit?* New York: Routledge, 187–203.

Mansfield, L. and Rich, E. (2013) 'Public health pedagogy, border crossings and physical activity at every size', *Critical Public Health*, 23(2): 356–370.

Maron, B., Carney, K., Lever, H., Lewis, J., Barac, I., Casey, S. and Sherrid, M. (2003) 'Relationship of race to sudden cardiac death in competitive athletes with hypertrophic cardiomyopathy', *Journal of the American College of Cardiology*, 41(6): 974–980.

Marshall, S. and Spencer, R. (2001) 'Concussion in rugby: the hidden epidemic', *Journal of Athletic Training*, 36(3): 334–338.

Martin, G. and Finn, R. (2011) 'Patients as team members: opportunities, challenges and paradoxes of including patients in multi-professional healthcare teams', *Sociology of Health and Illness*, 33(7): 1050–1065.

McClaren, P. (1996) *A Study of Injuries Sustained in Sport and Recreation in Ontario*. Unpublished Report for the Ontario Ministry of Citizenship, Culture and Recreation.

McCrea, M., Hammeke, T., Olsen, G. Leo, P. and Guskiewicz, K. (2004) 'Unreported concussion in high school football players: implications for prevention', *Clinical Journal of Sports Medicine*, 14: 13–17.

McCrory, P. (1999) 'You can run by you can't hide: the role of concussion severity scales in sport', *British Journal of Sports Medicine*, 33: 297–280.

McCrory, P. (2001a) 'When to retire after concussion?', *British Journal of Sports Medicine*, 35: 81–82.

McCrory, P. (2001b) 'Do mouthguards prevent concussion?', *British Journal of Sports Medicine*, 35: 380–382.

McCrory, P., Johnston, K., Meeuwisse, W., Aubry, M., Cantu, R., Dvorak, J., Graf-Baumann, T., Kelly, J., Lovell, M. and Schamasch, P. (2005) 'Summary and agreement statement of the 2nd International Conference on Concussion in Sport, Prague 2004', *British Journal of Sports Medicine*, 39: 196–204.

McCrory, P., Meeuwisse, W. Aubrey, M. *et al.* (2013) 'Consensus statement on concussion in sport: the 4th International Conference on Concussion in Sport held in Zurich, November 2012', *British Journal of Sports Medicine*, 47: 250–258.

McCutcheon, T., Curtis, J. and White, P. (1997) 'The socio-economic distribution of sport injuries: multivariate analyses using Canadian national data', *Sociology of Sport Journal*, 14: 57–72.

McEwan, I. and Taylor, W. (2010) ' "When do I get to run on with the magic sponge?" The twin illusions of meritocracy and democracy in the professions of sports medicine and physiotherapy', *Qualitative Research in Sport, Exercise and Health*, 2(1): 77–91.

McGannon, K., Cunningham, S. and Schinke, R. (2013) 'Understanding concussion in socio-cultural context: a media analysis of a National Hockey League star's concussion', *Psychology of Sport and Exercise*, 14: 891–899.

McKinlay, J. and Marceau, L. (2002) 'The end of the golden age of doctoring', *International Journal of Health Services*, 32(2): 379–416.

McNamee, M. and Partridge, B. (2013) 'Concussion in sports medicine ethics: policy, epistemic and ethical problems', *Sports Medicine and Ethics*, 13(10): 15–17.

McNamee, M., Partridge, B. and Anderson, L. (2015) 'Concussion in sport: conceptual and ethical issues', *Kinesiology Review*, 4: 190–202.

McNamee, M., Partridge, B. and Anderson, L. (2016) 'Concussion ethics and sports medicine', *Clinics in Sports Medicine*, 35(2): 257–268.

Menafoglio, A., Di Valentino, M., Segatto, J.-M., Sirgusa, P., Pezzolis, R., Maggi, M., Romano, G.A., Moschovistis, G. and Gallino, A. (2013) 'Cardiovascular screening in young athletes: controversies and feasibility', *Cardiovascular Medicine*, 16(1): 11–19.

Mennell, S. (1998) *Norbert Elias: An Introduction.* Oxford: Blackwell.

Milne, C. (2011) 'Practising sports and exercise medicine in an environment of rising medical costs', *British Journal of Sports Medicine*, 45: 945–946.

Mitchell, R., Finch, C. and Bourfous, S. (2010) 'Counting organised sport injury cases: evidence of incomplete capture from routine hospital collections', *Journal of Science and Medicine in Sport*, 13: 304–308.

Monaghan, L. (2001) *Bodybuilding, Drugs and Risk.* London: Routledge.

Monaghan, L. and Gabe, J. (2015) 'Chronic illness as biographical contingency? Young people's experiences of asthma', *Sociology of Health and Illness*, 37(8): 1236–1253.

Moore, L., Frost, J. and Britten, N. (2015) 'Context and complexity: the meaning of self-management for older adults with heart disease', *Sociology of Health and Illness*, 37(8): 1254–1269.

Morden, A., Jinks, C. and Ong, B.N (2015) 'Risk and self-managing chronic joint pain: looking beyond individual lifestyles and behaviour', *Sociology of Health and Illness*, 37(6): 888–903.

Moynihan, R. and Smith, R. (2002) 'Too much medicine? Almost certainly', *British Medical Journal*, 324: 859–860.

Mueller, F., Cantu, R. and van Camp, S. (1996) *Catastrophic Injuries in High School and College Sport.* Champaign, IL: Human Kinetics.

Müller, A. (2012) 'Pre-participation screenings in sports: a review of current genetic/nongenetic testing strategies', in D. Malcolm and P. Safai (eds), *The Social Organization of Sports Medicine*. New York: Routledge, 285–303.

Mummery, W.K., Schofield, G. and Spence, J.C. (2002) 'The epidemiology of medically attended sport and recreation injuries in Queensland', *Journal of Science and Medicine in Sport*, 5(4): 307–320.

Murphy, A.W., Martyn, C., Plunkett, P.K. and O'Connor, P. (1992) 'Sports injuries and the accident emergency department – ten years on', *Irish Medical Journal*, 85(1): 30–33.

Murray, S. (2008) 'Pathologizing "fatness": medical authority and popular culture', *Sociology of Sport Journal*, 25(1): 7–21.

Naci, H. and Ioannidis, J. (2013) 'Comparative effectiveness of exercise and drug interventions on mortality outcomes: metaepidemiological study', *British Medical Journal*, 347: f5577.

Naidoo, J. and Wills, J. (1994) *Health Promotion: Foundations for Practice*. London: Baillière Tindall.

Nancarrow, S. and Borthwick, A.M. (2005) 'Dynamic professional boundaries in the healthcare workforce', *Sociology of Health & Illness*, 27(7): 897–919.

Nettleton, S. (2006) *The Sociology of Health and Illness* (2nd edn). Cambridge, UK: Polity.

Nettleton, S. and Bunton, R. (1995) 'Sociological critiques of health promotion', in R. Bunton, S. Nettleton and R. Burrows (eds), *The Sociology of Health Promotion: Critical Analyses of Consumption, Lifestyle and Risk*. London: Routledge, 39–56.

Nettleton, S. and Hardey, M. (2006) 'Running away with health: the urban marathon and the construction of "charitable bodies"', *Health*, 10(4): 441–460.

Neville, R. (2012) 'Considering a complemental model of health and fitness', *Sociology of Health and Illness*, 35(3): 479–492.

Neville, R. (2013) 'Exercise is medicine: some cautionary remarks in principle as well as in practice', *Medicine and Health Care Philosophy*, 16(3): 615–622.

Nicholl, J.P., Coleman, P., Brazier, J. (1994) 'Health and healthcare costs and benefits of exercise', *Pharmacoeconomics*, 5(2): 109–122.

Nicholl, J.P., Coleman, P. and Williams, B.T. (1995) 'The epidemiology of sports and exercise related injury in the United Kingdom', *British Journal of Sports Medicine*, 29(4): 232–238.

Nicholls, D.A. and Cheek, J. (2006) 'Physiotherapy and the shadow of prostitution: the Society of Trained Masseuses and the massage scandals of 1894', *Social Science and Medicine*, 62: 2236–2348.

Nike (2012) *Designed to Move: A Physical Activity Action Agenda*. www.designedtomove.org/resources/designed-to-move-report. Accessed 20 April 2016.

Nixon, H.L. II (1992) 'A social network analysis of influences on athletes to play with pain and injuries', *Journal of Sport and Social Issues*, 16: 127–135.

O'Halloran, P., Tzortziou Brown, V., Morgan, K., Maffulli, N., Perry, M. and Morrissey, D. (2009) 'The role of the sports and exercise medicine physician in the national health service', *British Journal of Sports Medicine*, 45:e1 doi:10.1136/bjsm.2010.081554.62.

Overbye, M. and Wagner, U. (2013) 'Experiences, attitudes and trust: an inquiry into elite athletes' perception of the whereabouts reporting system', *International Journal of Sport Policy and Politics*, 6(3): 407–428.

Owen, R. (2012) 'London 2012: Physios report Olympics injury "legacy"', www.bbc.co.uk/news/uk-wales-19560103. Accessed 12 May 2016.

Pampel, F. (2012) 'Does reading keep you thin? Leisure activities, cultural tastes, and body weight in comparative perspective', *Sociology of Health and Illness*, 34(3): 396–411.

Papadakis, M., Whyte, G. and Sharma, S. (2008) 'Preparticipation screening for cardiovascular abnormalities in young competitive athletes', *British Medical Journal*, 337: 806–811.

Park, J. (2005) 'Governing doped bodies: the World Anti-Doping Agency and the global culture of surveillance', *Cultural Studies <=> Critical Methodologies*, 5(2): 174–188.

Park, R. (2015) *Gender, Sport, Science: Selected writings of Roberta J. Park* (edited by J.A. Mangan and P. Vertinsky). Abingdon: Routledge.

Parry, R. (2009) 'Practitioners' accounts for treatment actions and recommendations in physiotherapy: when do they occur, how are they structured, what do they do?' *Sociology of Health and Illness*, 31(6): 835–853.

Parsons, T. (1975) 'The sick role and the role of the physician reconsidered', *The Milbank Memorial Fund Quarterly*, 53(3): 257–278.

Partridge, B. (2014) 'Dazed and confused: sports medicine, conflicts of interest, and concussion management', *Bioethical Inquiry*, 11: 65–74.

Partridge, B. and Hall, W. (2014) 'Repeated head injuries in Australia's collision sports highlight ethical and evidential gaps in concussion management policies', *Neuroethics*, 8(1): 39–45.

Petersen, A. and Lupton, D. (1996) *The New Public Health: Discourses, Knowledges, Strategies*. London: Sage.

Pfeffer, N. (2004) 'Screening for breast cancer: candidacy and compliance', *Social Science and Medicine*, 58: 151–160.

Pfister, G. (2011) ' "Sports" medicine in Germany and its struggle for professional status', *Canadian Bulletin of Medical History*, 28(2): 271–292.

PHE (2014) *Everybody Active, Everyday: An Evidence Based Approach to Physical Activity*. London: Public Health England.

Phillips, E.M., Capell, J. and Jonas, S. (2009a) 'Staying active', in S. Jonas, and E. Philips (eds) *ACSM's Exercise is Medicine: A Clinician's Guide to Exercise Prescription*. Philadelphia: Lippincott, Williams and Wilkins, 134–150.

Phillips, E.M., Capell, J. and Jonas, S. (2009b) 'Getting started as a regular exerciser'. In S. Jonas, and E. Philips (eds), *ACSM's Exercise is Medicine: A Clinician's Guide to Exercise Prescription*. Philadelphia: Lippincott, Williams and Wilkins, 84–98.

Pierret, J. (2003) 'The illness experience: state of knowledge and perspectives for research', *Sociology of Health and Illness*, 25: 4–22.

Piggin, J. (2014) 'Designed to move? Physical activity lobbying and the politics of productivity', *Health Education Journal*, 74(1): 16–27.

Piggin, J. and Bairner, A. (2016) 'The global physical inactivity pandemic: an analysis of knowledge production', *Sport, Education and Society*, 21(2): 131–147.

Pike, E. (2005). 'Doctors just say "rest and take ibuprofen": a critical examination of the role of "non-orthodox" health care in women's sport', *International Review for the Sociology of Sport*, 40(3): 201–219.

Pilnick, A. (2008) ' "It's something for you both to think about": choice and decision making in nuchal translucency screening for Down's syndrome', *Sociology of Health and Illness*, 30(4): 511–530.

Pollit, R. (2006) 'International perspectives on newborn screening', *Journal of Inherited Metabolic Disease*, 29: 390–396.

Pollock, A. (2014) *Tackling Rugby: What Every Parent Should Know about Injuries*. Verso: London.

Pollock, A. and Kirkwood, G. (2008) *Response to the Scottish Government's Consultation on 'Glasgow 2014 – Delivering a Lasting Legacy for Scotland'*. Edinburgh: Centre for International Public Health Policy.

Popay, J., Whitehead, M. and Hunter, D. (2010) 'Editorial: injustice is killing people on a large scale – but what is to be done about it', *Journal of Public Health*, 32(2): 148–149.

Porter, D. (1999) *Health, Civilization and the State: A History of Public Health from Ancient to Modern Times*. Routledge.

Price, J., Malliaras, P. and Hudson, Z. (2012) 'Current practices in determining return to play following head injury in professional football in the UK', *British Journal of Sports Medicine*, 46: 1000–1003.

Prior, L. (2003) 'Belief, knowledge and expertise: the emergence of the lay expert in medical sociology', *Sociology of Health and Illness*, 25 (Silver Anniversary Issue): 41–57.

Prior, L., Scott, D., Hunter, R., Donnelly, M., Tully, M., Cupples, M. and Kee, F. (2014) 'Exploring lay views on physical activity and their implications for public health policy. A case study from East Belfast', *Social Science and Medicine*, 114: 73–80.

Rafalovich, A. (2005) 'Exploring clinician uncertainty in the diagnosis and treatment of Attention Deficit Hyperactivity Disorder', *Sociology of Health and Illness*, 27: 305–323.

RCP (1991) *Medical Aspects of Exercise: Benefits and Risks*. London: Royal College of Physicians.

RCP (2012) *Exercise for Life: Physical Activity in Health and Disease. Recommendations of the Sport and Exercise Medicine Committee Working Party of the Royal College of Physicians*. London: Royal College of Physicians.

Reid, C., Stewart, E. and Thorne, G. (2004) 'Multidisciplinary sport science teams in elite sport: comprehensive servicing or conflict and confusion?' *The Sports Psychologist*, 18: 204–217.

Reynolds, L.A. and Tansey, E.M. (eds) (2009) *The Development of Sports Medicine in Twentieth Century Britain*. London: Wellcome Trust Centre.

Riordan, J. (1987) 'Sports medicine in the Soviet Union and German Democratic Republic', *Social Science and Medicine*, 25(1): 19–28.

Roderick, M. (2006) *The Work of Professional Football*. London: Routledge.

Roderick, M., Waddington, I. and Parker, G. (2000) 'Playing hurt: managing injuries in English professional football', *International Review for the Sociology of Sport*, 35: 165–180.

Rose, G. (1981) 'Strategy of prevention: lessons from cardiovascular disease', *British Medical Journal*, 282: 1847–1851.

Rowell, S. and Rees-Jones, A. (1988) 'Injuries treated at a sports injury clinic compared with a neighbouring accident and emergency department', *British Journal of Sports Medicine*, (22): 157–160.

RunningUSA (2014) '2014 annual marathon report', www.runningusa.org/index.cfm?fuseaction=news.details&ArticleId=332. Accessed 18 May 2016.

Ryan, A.J. (1989) 'Sports medicine in the world today', in A.J. Ryan and F.L. Allman (eds), *Sports Medicine*. San Diego: Academic Press, 3–13.

Safai, P. (2003) 'Healing the body in the "culture of risk": examining the negotiations of treatment between sport medicine clinicians and injured athletes in Canadian intercollegiate sport', *Sociology of Sport Journal*, 20(2): 127–146.

Safai, P. (2005) 'The demise of the Sport Medicine and Science Council of Canada', *Sport History Review*, 36: 91–114.

Safai, P. (2007) 'A critical analysis of the development of sport medicine in Canada, 1955–1980', *International Review for the Sociology of Sport*, 42(3): 321–341.

Safai, P. (2008) 'Sport and health', in B. Houlihan (ed.), *Sport and Society: A Student Introduction* (2nd edn). London: Sage, 155–172.

Saks, M. (1995) *Professions and the Public Interest: Medical Power, Altruism and Alternative Medicine*. London: Routledge.

Sallis, R.E. (2009) 'Exercise is medicine and physicians need to prescribe it!' *British Journal of Sports Medicine*, 43(1): 3–4.

Sanchez Garcia, R. and Malcolm, D. (2010) 'De-civilizing, civilizing or informalizing? The international development of mixed martial arts', *International Review of the Sociology of Sport*, 45(1): 1–20.

Sandelin, J., Kiviluoto, O., Santavirta, S. and Honkanen, R. (1985) 'Outcome of sports injuries treated in a casualty department', *British Journal of Sports Medicine*, 19(2): 103–106.

Sanders, T. and Harrison, S. (2008) 'Professional legitimacy claims in the multidisciplinary workplace: the case of heart failure care', *Sociology of Health & Illness*, 30(2): 289–308.

Sanderson, T., Calnan, M., Morris, M., Richards, P. and Hewlett, S. (2011) 'Shifting normalities: interactions of changing conceptions of a normal life and the normalisation of symptoms in rheumatoid arthritis', *Sociology of Health and Illness*, 33(4): 618–633.

Sassatelli, R. (2000) 'The commercialization of discipline: keep-fit culture and its values', *Journal of Modern Italian Studies*, 5(3): 396–411.

Satterthwaite, P., Norton, R., Larmer, P. and Robinson, E. (1999) 'Risk factors for injuries and other health problems sustained in a marathon', *British Journal of Sports Medicine*, 33(1): 22–26.

Saukko, P., Farrimond, H., Evans, P. and Qureshi, N. (2012) 'Beyond beliefs: risk assessment technologies shaping patients' experiences of heart disease prevention', *Sociology of Health and Illness*, 34(4): 560–575.

Scambler, G. (2005) *Sport and Society: History, Power and Culture*. Maidenhead: Open University Press.

Scambler, G., Ohlsson, S. and Griva, K. (2004) 'Sport, health and identity: social and cultural change in disorganised capitalism', in D. Kelleher and G. Leavey (eds), *Identity and Health*. London: Routledge, 99–102.

Scarborough, P., Bhatnagar, P., Wickramasinghe, K., Allender, S., Foster, C. and Rayner, M. (2011) 'The economic burden of ill health due to diet, physical inactivity, smoking, alcohol and obesity in the UK: an update to 2006–07 NHS costs', *Journal of Public Health*, 33(4): 527–535.

Sceats, J. and Gilles, J. (1989) 'Paediatric attendance at Waikato Hospital accident and emergency department 1980–86', *New Zealand Medical Journal*, 102: 467–469.

Schneider, S., Seither, B., Tonges, S and Schmitt, H. (2006) 'Sports injuries: population based representative data on incidence, diagnosis, sequelae, and high risk groups', *British Journal of Sports Medicine*, 40: 334–339.

Schwarz, A. (2011) 'A case against helmets in lacrosse', *New York Times*, 16 February 2011, www.nytimes.com/2011/02/17/sports/17lacrosse.html?_r=0. Accessed 23 March 2016.

Scott, A. (2010) '*"More professional?" The Occupational Practices of Sports Medicine Clinicians Working with British Olympic athletes*. Unpublished PhD thesis, Loughborough University, Loughborough, UK.

Scott, A. (2012) 'Sport and exercise medicine's professional project: the impact of formal qualifications on the organization of British Olympic medical services', *International Review for the Sociology of Sport*, 49(5): 575–591.

Scott, Andy (2012) 'All footballers should have a cardiac certificate', *Guardian*, 19 March, www.theguardian.com/football/2012/mar/19/abrice-muamba-andy-scott-football-heart-screening. Accessed 16 April 2016.

Scott, A. and Malcolm, D. (2015) ' "Involved in every step": how working practices shape the influence of physiotherapists in elite sport', *Qualitative Research in Sport, Exercise and Health*, 7(4–5): 539–557.

Sen, A. (2002) 'Health: perception versus observation', *British Medical Journal*, 324: 860–861.

Sheard, K. (1998) ' "Brutal and degrading": the medical profession and boxing, 1838–1984', *International Journal of the History of Sport*, 15(3): 74–102.

Shilling, C. (1993) *The Body and Social Theory*. London: Sage.

Sluggett, B. (2011) 'Sport's doping game: surveillance in the biotech age', *Sociology of Sport Journal*, 28: 387–403.

Smith, S.L. (1998) 'Athletes, runners, and joggers: participant-group dynamics in a sport of "individuals" ', *Sociology of Sport Journal*, 15: 174–192.

Smith, A. and Green, K. (2006) 'The place of sport and physical activity in young people's lives and its implications for health: some sociological comments', *Journal of Youth Studies*, 8(2): 241–253.

Smith-Maguire, J. (2008) *Fit for Consumption: Sociology and the Business of Fitness*. London: Routledge.

Sparkes, A. and Smith, B. (2002) 'Men, sport, spinal chord injury and the construction of coherence: narrative practice in action', *Qualitative Research*, 2(2): 143–171.

Sport England (2012) *Satisfaction with the Quality of the Sporting Experience Survey (SQSE 4): Drop Out Survey Report*. London: Sport England.

Steinvil, A., Chundadze, T., Zeltser, D., Rogowski, O., Halkin, A., Galily, Y., Perluk, H. and Viskin, S. (2011) 'Mandatory electrocardiographic screening of athletes to reduce their risk of sudden death: proven fact or wishful thinking?' *Journal of the American College of Cardiology*, 57(11): 1291–1296.

Stovitz, S.D. and Satin, D.J. (2006) 'Professionalism and the ethics of the sideline physician', *Current Sports Medicine Reports*, 5: 120–124.

Stuij, M. (2011) 'Explaining trends in body weight: Offers' rational and myopic choice vs Elias' theory of civilising processes', *Social History of Medicine*, 243: 796–812.

Suddick, K.M. and De Souza, L. (2006) 'Therapists' experiences and perceptions of teamwork in neurological rehabilitation: reasoning behind the team approach, structure and composition of the team and teamworking processes', *Physiotherapy Research International*, 11(2): 72–83.

Symons, J. (2016) 'From wearing corn plasters on your nipples to having sex beforehand, experts reveal how to ensure you got to the start – and finish – of the London Marathon'. Mailonline, 19 April 2016. www.dailymail.co.uk/health/article-3538155/From-wearing-corn-plasters-nipples-having-sex-experts-reveal-ensure-start-finish-London-Marathon.html. Accessed 20 April 2016.

Testoni, D., Hornik, C., Smith, P.B., Benjamin, D.K. and McKinney, R.E. (2013) 'Sports medicine and ethics', *The American Journal of Bioethics*, 13(10): 4–12.

Theberge, N. (2000) *Higher Goals: Women's Ice Hockey and the Politics of Gender*. New York: SUNY Press.

Theberge, N. (2007) ' "It's not about health, it's about performance". Sport medicine, health and the culture of risk in Canadian sport', in J. Hargreaves and P. Vertinsky (eds), *Physical Culture, Power and the Body*. London: Routledge, 176–194.

Theberge, N. (2008) 'The integration of chiropractors into healthcare teams: a case study from sports medicine', *Sociology of Health and Illness*, 30(1): 19–34.

Theberge, N. (2009a) ' "We have all the bases covered". Constructions of professional boundaries in sport medicine', *International Review for the Sociology of Sport*, 44(2): 265–282.

Theberge, N. (2009b) 'Professional identities and the practice of sport medicine in Canada: a comparative analysis of two sporting contexts', on J. Harris. and A. Parker (eds), *Sport and Social Identities*. Basingstoke: Palgrave Macmillan, 49–69.

Theberge, N. (2012) 'Challenges to the implementation of a rationalized model of sports medicine: an analysis in the Canadian context', in D. Malcolm and P. Safai (eds), *The Social Organization of Sports Medicine: Critical Socio-cultural Perspectives*. New York: Routledge, 164–185.

Theodoraki, E. (1999) 'The making of the UK Sports Institute', *Managing Leisure*, 4: 187–200.

Thing, L. (2012) 'Docile bodies or reflexive users? On the individualization of medical risk in sports', in D. Malcolm and P. Safai (eds), *The Social Organization of Sports Medicine: Critical Socio-Cultural Perspectives*. New York: Routledge, 187–203.

Thornquist, E. (1995) 'Musculoskeletal suffering: diagnosis and a variant view', *Sociology of Health and Illness*, 17(2): 166–192.

Thorpe, O., Johnston, K. and Kumar, S. (2012) 'Barriers and enablers to physical activity participation in patients with COPD', *Journal of Cardiopulmonary Rehabilitation and Prevention*, 32: 359–369.

Timmermans, S. (2013) 'Seven warrants for qualitative health sociology', *Social Science and Medicine*, 77: 1–8.

Timmermans, S. and Buchbinder, M. (2012) 'Expanded newborn screening: articulating the ontology of diseases with bridging work in the clinic', *Sociology of Health and Illness*, 34(2): 208–220.

Tunstall Pedoe, D. (no date) 'London Marathon: what we know about the incidence of injury, illness and death in the London Marathon'. www.pponline.co.uk/encyc/london-marathon-what-we-know-about-the-incidence-of-injury-illness-and-death-in-the-london-marathon-881. Accessed 6 July 2013.

Turner, B.S. (1995) *Medical Power and Social Knowledge* (2nd edn). London: Sage.

UKactive (2014) *Turning the Tide of Inactivity*. London: UKactive.

van der Sluis, C.K., Eisma, W.H., Groothoff, J.W., and ten Duis, H.J. (1998) 'Long-term physical, psychological and social consequences of severe injuries', *Injury*, 29(4): 281–285.

van Krieken, R. (1998) *Norbert Elias*. London: Routledge.

van Mechelen, W., Hlobil, H. and Kemper, H.C. (1992) 'Incidence, severity, aetiology and prevention of sports injuries: a review of concepts', *Sports Medicine*, 14(2): 82–99.

Veblen, T. (1899) *The Theory of the Leisure Class: An Economic Study of Institutions*. New York, Macmillan.

Vertinsky, P. (1990) *The Eternally Wounded Woman: Women, Doctors and Exercise in the Late Nineteenth Century*. Manchester: Manchester University Press.

Waddington, I. (1996) 'The development of sports medicine', *Sociology of Sport Journal*, 13(2): 176–196.

Waddington, I. (2000) *Sport, Health and Drugs: A Critical Sociological Investigation*. London: E & FN Spon.

Waddington, I. (2002) 'Jobs for the boys? A study of the employment of club doctors and physiotherapists in English professional football', *Soccer & Society*, 3(1): 51–64.

Waddington, I. (2012) 'Sports medicine, client control and the limits of professional autonomy', in D. Malcolm and P. Safai (eds), *The Social Organization of Sports Medicine: Critical Socio-cultural Perspectives*. New York: Routledge, 204–226.

Waddington, I. and Murphy, P. (1992) 'Drugs, sport and ideologies', in E. Dunning and C. Rojek (eds), *Sport and Leisure in the Civilizing Process*. London: Macmillan, 36–64.

Waddington, I. and Smith, A. (2009) *An Introduction to Drugs in Sport: Addicted to Winning?* London: Routledge.

Waddington, I., Roderick, M. and Naik, R. (2001) 'Methods of appointment and qualifications of club doctors and physiotherapists in English professional football: some problems and issues', *British Journal of Sports Medicine*, 35: 48–53.

Wagstaff, C., Gilmore, S. and Thelwell, R. (2015) 'Sport medicine and sport science practitioners' experiences of organizational change', *Scandinavian Journal of Medicine and Science in Sports*, 25(5): 685–698.

Walk, S. (1997) 'Peers in pain: the experiences of student athletic trainers', *Sociology of Sport Journal*, 14(1): 22–56.

Walk, S. (2004) 'Athletic trainers: between care and social control', in K. Young (ed.), *Sporting Bodies, Damaged Selves*. Oxford: Elsevier, 251–267.

Waring, J. and Bishop, S. (2010) 'Lean healthcare: rhetoric, ritual and resistance', *Social Science & Medicine*, 71(7): 1332–1340.

Watters, D.A.K., Brooks, S., Elton, R.A. and Little, K. (1984) 'Sports injuries in an accident and emergency department', *Archives of Emergency Medicine*, 2: 105–112.

Weaver, N., Spicer, R., Marshall, S. and Muller, F. (1999) 'Cost of athletic injuries in 12 North Carolina high school sports', *Medicine and Science in Sports and Exercise*, 31(5): S93.

Webb, J. (2014) 'Sports concussion "breathalyser" proposed', 11 September 2014, www.bbc.co.uk/news/science-environment-29146654. Accessed 23 March 2016.

Welshman, J. (1998) 'Only connect: the history of sport, medicine and society', *International Journal of the History of Sport*, 15(2): 1–21.

White, P. (2004) 'The costs of injury from sport, exercise and physical activity: a review of the evidence', in K. Young (ed.), *Sporting Bodies, Damaged Selves*. Oxford: Elsevier.

WHO (2003) *Health and Development through Physical Activity and Sport*. Geneva: World Health Organization.

WHO (2011) *Promoting Sport and Enhancing Health in European Union Countries: A Policy Content Analysis to Support Action*. Copenhagen: World Health Organization (Europe).

WHO (2012) *Global Recommendations on Physical Activity and Health*. Geneva: World Health Organization.

Wilkinson, M. and Marmot, R. (eds) (2003) *The Social Determinants of Health*. Oxford: Oxford University Press.

Williams, G. and Popay, J. (1994) 'Lay knowledge and the privilege of experience', in J. Gabe, D. Kelleher and G. Williams (eds), *Challenging Medicine*. London: Routledge, 118–139.

Williams, J. (2011) 'The challenge of increasing uptake of pulmonary rehabilitation: what can we do to maximize the chances of success?', *Chronic Respiratory Disease*, 8(2): 87–88.

Williams, J. and Sperryn, P. (eds) (1976) *Sports Medicine* (2nd ed.). London: Edward Arnold.

Williams, J.G.P. (1979) 'The Federation Internationale de Medicine Sportive', *British Journal of Sports Medicine*, 13: 180–181.

Williams, S.J. (1993) *Chronic Respiratory Illness*. London: Routledge.

Williams, S.J. (2000) 'Chronic illness as biographical disruption or biographical disruption as chronic illness? Reflections on a core concept', *Sociology of Health and Illness*, 22(1): 40–67.

Williams, S.J., Martin, P. and Gabe, J. (2011) 'The pharmaceuticalisation of society? A framework for analysis', *Sociology of Health and Illness*, 33(5): 710–725.

Williams, V., Bruton, A., Ellis-Hill, C. and McPherson, K. (2011) 'The importance of movement for people living with chronic obstructive pulmonary disease', *Qualitative Health Research*, 21(9): 1239–1248.

Wilson, J. and Jungner, G. (1968) *Principles and Practice of Screening for Disease*. Geneva: World Health Organization.

Wrynn, A. (2004) 'The human factor: science, medicine and the International Olympic Committee', *Sport and Society*, 7(2): 211–231.

Yair, G. (2007) 'Existential uncertainty and the will to conform: the expressive basis of Coleman's rational choice paradigm', *Sociology*, 41: 681–698.

Young, K. (1993) 'Violence, risk and liability in male sports culture', *Sociology of Sport Journal*, 10(4): 373–396.

Zola, I. (1972) 'Medicine as an institution of social control', *Sociological Review*, 20(4): 487–504.

Zola, I. (1983) *Socio-medical Inquiries*. Philadelphia: Temple Press.

Index

Milton Keynes UK
Ingram Content Group UK Ltd.
UKHW031149141024
449569UK00024B/955